Customer Service in Health Care

A Grassroots Approach to Creating a Culture of Service Excellence

Kristin Baird

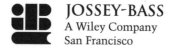

JOSSEY-BASS
A Wiley Company
San Francisco

Published by Jossey-Bass
A Wiley Imprint
989 Market Street, San Francisco, CA 94103-1741   www.josseybass.com

Jossey-Bass books and products are available through most bookstores. To contact Jossey-Bass directly call our Customer Care Department within the U.S. at 800-956-7739, outside the U.S. at 317-572-3986, or fax 317-572-4002.

Jossey-Bass also publishes its books in a variety of electronic formats. Some content that appears in print may not be available in electronic books.

Cover design by Dan Stein

Library of Congress Cataloging-in-Publication Data

Baird, Kristin.
    Customer service in health care : a grassroots approach to creating a culture of service excellence / by Kristin Baird.
       p.   cm.
    Includes index.
    ISBN 1-55648-269-8 (pbk.)
    Reprint ISBN 0-7879-5251-6
    1. Medical care—Customer services. 2. Patient satisfaction.
I. Title.
    [DNLM: 1. Health Services—standards. 2. Patient Satisfaction.
W 85 B162c 1999]
R7727.B276   1999
362.1'068—dc21
DNLM/DLC
for Library of Congress   99-36797

Printed in the United States of America
FIRST EDITION
PB Printing   10 9 8 7 6 5

Contents

List of Figures and Tables

Figures

Tables

About the Author

Kristin Baird has been in health care since 1977. She is currently vice president of business development and marketing for Watertown (WI) Area Health Services and president of Baird Consulting, Inc. Ms. Baird's expertise in health care marketing and communications began as a clinician and freelance writer. Her experience as a registered nurse, marketer, administrator, and consultant has shaped a keen understanding of customer service from a variety of perspectives. Her interest and expertise in customer service stems from practical, on-the-job experience as well as research.

An experienced focus group facilitator, speaker, and trainer, Ms. Baird has given speeches and seminars on health care marketing, communication, and customer service to dozens of groups in a variety of health care settings.

Ms. Baird holds a bachelor of science degree in nursing and a master's degree in health services administration.

Preface

Have you ever stood in the checkout line at the grocery store and been caught up in the magazine headlines for the dozens of diets claiming to melt pounds off you like butter in the sun? "Try this and you'll lose anywhere from 10 pounds in one week to 50 pounds in a month!" I have to admit that more than once I have picked up those magazines in the hope of finding the quick fix. Maybe this one would be the magic bullet. Maybe it's easier than I thought. However, anyone who has battled with weight problems will tell you that fad diets won't work. What does work is a lifelong commitment to a healthy, well-balanced diet, moderation, and regular exercise. This isn't rocket science. But knowing this information and living it are two very different things. Sitting on your sofa reading about fitness and nutrition will only improve your mind. In order to set a change into motion, you need to apply that knowledge into action.

Creating a culture of service excellence is very similar to living a healthy, well-balanced life. This book can't make a tabloid-style promise of an organizational turnaround in 30 days or less. It does, however, present the fundamentals essential to changing attitudes and improving performance that will bring individuals closer to the organization's mission and, in turn, in step with specific values and standards. Like any lifestyle change, a lasting organizational change requires knowledge, vigilance, goal setting, perseverance, and the ability to recognize and reward progress. But, above all, it requires a strong desire to change that is founded in a core belief that it is the right thing to do—for the patient, the employee, the physicians, and the public that you serve.

Slapping together a reward program or customer service training program without linking it to standards and core philosophies would be like getting liposuction to cure obesity. You may look better on the surface for a while, but the erosion of the internal systems will eventually kill you. Cosmetic or superficial changes won't alter the core of customer service.

This book is like a blueprint and action plan for remodeling. It will help you to check the foundation, reinforce the support beams, and then start remodeling. The foundation is what your organization stands for. It is the mission and the history that were there at the inception. The support beams are the middle management that will either give the structure stability or hasten a collapse. And, finally, the walls, floors, and fixtures are the line employees who make the finished product.

Figure 2-1 in chapter 2 outlines a road map for success. Presented as a storyboard/flowchart, the road map provides a visual schematic to follow on your journey toward customer service excellence. The diagram demonstrates that building a culture of service excellence takes commitment at all levels of the organization. Like any new habit, practicing customer service excellence doesn't feel natural at first and often feels downright uncomfortable.

This book is written based on personal experiences. There are several citations from reliable researchers in the field, but the core content is based on my 20 years of experience in a variety of health care settings ranging from nursing homes and rural hospitals to large integrated systems. My perspective includes experience as a nurse assistant, an RN, a nurse manager, marketing and public relations director, consultant, and administrator. It was from this variety of past experience that I drew when introducing a customer service program at Watertown Memorial Hospital in 1997. As an organization, we are still growing and improving in the area of customer service, which is as it should be. The real work is never finished in customer service. If you want a quick fix or a one-shot training session, this book is not for you. You will only benefit from one or two chapters. If, however, you are willing to take a critical look at your organization, core values, and commitment to the well-being of customers, staff, and community, this book will provide you with a wealth of ideas and inspiration.

Health care is really the only profession rooted in a history of healing bodies, minds, and spirits. From its very beginnings and throughout recorded history, health care providers have been servants with a mission of healing. As we evolved, however, we became caught up in the science of medicine, technology, and pharmacology; and miracle drugs, state-of-the-art surgical techniques, and powerful imaging technology helped to foster the scientific focus. Simultaneously, we were becoming big business. We focused more on the cash flow, market share, and financial ratios and, in doing so, allowed the human elements of health care to slip through our fingers. Our role as true servants or, in modern vernacular, service-minded individuals was lost or at least misplaced. It's time to take it back. It's time to reclaim our role in society as the truest of servants. Then and only then will we be fulfilling the needs of our communities.

Acknowledgments

How does a busy mother of three manage to complete a book on deadline while juggling a full-time job and consulting? I had a lot of encouragement and support from colleagues who were willing to review my work and offer honest feedback. For that, I thank Jan Triplett, Sheila Murphy, John Kosanovich, Tom Peterson, Dr. Thom McGorey, Mark Dziewior and the customer service team of Watertown Area Health Services, and Dr. Michael Grajewsky. There were several individuals who shared their professional experience in building customer service programs. I thank Marsha Borling, Quint Studer, and Bob Richards for sharing their insights and experience with me. But perhaps the people who have helped influence me the most, both in my life and as the author of this book, are those who have helped to rekindle my passion for service. They include the late Rev. Lloyd Werthmann, who helped me move service from a cerebral function to a spiritually growing experience; Quint Studer, who guided me in melding nursing with business development; and John Kosanovich and my colleagues at Watertown Area Health Services, who continue to teach me about patience and perseverance as we change and grow in our mission together.

CHAPTER ONE

Why Customer Service?

Objectives

After completing this chapter the reader will:

- Recognize customer service excellence as an essential component of business development

- Understand the financial repercussions of poor customer service

- Understand the levels of marketing achievement and the value of positive word of mouth

Before embarking on your journey toward a culture of service excellence, you will need to connect with your organization's leadership. The first step for every organization begins with the leadership. In order to have a successful program, leaders must have a solid understanding of, and respect for, the role of customer service.

This chapter presents the leadership team with background information that validates the need for organizationwide involvement and clear standards for performance. Until the senior leaders and middle managers believe in the value of customer service as it relates to the organization's mission and bottom line, there is little chance of shifting the corporate culture.

In many situations, the contents of this chapter will be like preaching to the choir. But even if that is the case, reviewing this information is important because it often creates a sense of urgency for the reader. "We know it's important, but where do we begin?" Only when this sense of urgency is created will the leadership be ready to move to the next level.

What Are the Standards of Behavior?

Be nice. Play fair. Share your toys. Don't fight. Do unto others as you would have them do unto you. Each of us receives a lifetime of messages directed at how we should interact with one another. Those lessons are learned at the dinner table, in the classroom, on the playground, and in Sunday school. Passed on through generations, they craft the ground rules of acceptable behavior in most social situations. However, these clichés give little, if any, clear directives about behavior. In fact, each is quite passive. They all imply: Don't make waves, keep quiet, and if you don't bother anyone, you'll get by. There is really no message about finding better ways to interact or proactively design your behavior.

The Golden Rule with a New Twist

Do unto others as you would have them do unto you? Or as they would like done unto them? Think about it: The golden rule implies that our desires are the same as others and, further, that we already know what they would like done unto them. If that were actually the case, marketing would be easy. We'd simply decide what we like or want, then pass it along to others. The reality is that patients know what they want, but more often than not we fail to ask and deliver on their requests.

Expectations Are Higher in Health Care

Playing a word association game has been a standard in my public speaking agenda. When talking with community groups about health care, I will say the word *hospital* and ask the audience to say the first word that comes to mind. In most cases, I hear words like *doctor, nurse, emergency, surgery,* or *high tech.* From their comments, one can see that there is a basic assumption about the level of competency found in a hospital or health care setting. I have never heard anyone respond with the words *housekeeping, maintenance, accounting,* or *dietary.* The response is always associated with professions that require extensive training and education. From this brief but telling exercise, I have come to believe that the public sees everyone involved in health care as a highly trained skilled professional. When they reach out to us for care, they lump all of us into one collective group called *the clinic* or *the hospital.* Their opinions are forming long before the x-ray is taken or the blood is drawn.

Health care, by its very nature, is a highly personal service. Our patients are expected to share their most intimate secrets, often with complete strangers. Not only do we ask them personal details about bodily functions, lifestyle habits, and mental status, we expect them to engage in these conversations openly and honestly while wearing nothing but a paper towel and socks. Worse yet, we ask them for the personal details over and over during a single encounter.

It's important for all health care workers to remember that in the vast majority of situations, our patients are coming to us because something is wrong. Even with the more recent push for wellness, our medical model has been built around people coming to hospitals and clinics when they are injured or ill. Some of life's most memorable events happen in and around health care settings. A traumatic accident, grim diagnosis, surgery, or the birth of a baby are life-changing events. I have yet to meet anyone who looks forward to an admission to an emergency room or hospital. When patients and their loved ones come in contact with hospitals and clinics, they are usually under emotional and physical stress. Emotions run high when people are under stress. If all health care employees can keep this in mind as they come into contact with patients, visitors, and other family members, they are much more likely to act with compassion and care.

In her introduction to the book *The Healthcare Customer Service Revolution,* Peggy Zimmerman states, "We have surveyed thousands of patients and interviewed dozens of employers throughout the country to get their reactions to their personal experiences in healthcare situations. They all confirm that what needs to be improved in the healthcare arena is the human element."[1]

Although it's affirming to read that others hold the same beliefs as I, all one has to do is think about his or her own expectations and the shortcomings encountered as health care consumers, and we'd all have a clearer understanding of the missing human element.

In the American Hospital Association's landmark study *Reality Check, Public Perceptions of Healthcare and Hospitals,* researchers reported that "the public feels a growing impact upon themselves and their families in terms of reduced access, higher cost, lower quality, the competence of care givers and a trend toward impersonal care. They see a growing focus on the financial 'bottom line' overwhelming what they believe should be a dedication to individual patient care."[2] Those words from the study's executive summary clarify the need for better, more personalized patient care. When each member of the health care team begins to take ownership for every encounter, then and only then will we begin to alter the public's perceptions of the health care profession.

This book presents a course of action each health care organization can take to improve customer service based on a pragmatic, grassroots approach. The word *customer* is used throughout the book because it encourages the reader to embrace a view of customer that includes more than just a patient receiving treatment. The goal of this book is to assist the reader to identify the various stakeholder groups known as customers both inside and outside the organization and to further define their unique needs and expectations.

The Direct and Indirect Costs of a Bad Experience

In a 1997 article, D. Zimmerman validated the need for improving customer service at all levels of health care.[3] The research targeted managed care organizations (MCOs), employers, patients, and hospitals to gain insights into customer satisfaction issues. The implications of the findings are significant. Surveys of 25 Fortune 500 companies representing millions of employees revealed that 60 percent of the employers survey their employees for satisfaction with providers and another 21 percent indicate that they plan to in the near future. More than 50 percent of the employers indicated that they would drop their current plan if customer service issues continued to be a problem.

The MCOs surveyed in the Zimmerman study represented over 25 million subscribers. All of the MCOs said that they are currently surveying members or plan to do so in the near future. Nearly 50 percent stated that they would drop providers who failed to meet customer service standards.

Also surveyed were 2,000 patients from 17 states who had been treated at over 30 hospitals and in hundreds of physicians' offices. Virtually all of them expressed some dissatisfaction with customer service. The research went on to define patient perception of service in terms of compassion, fast service, and friendliness.

Even though nearly one-third of the hospitals included in the Zimmerman research had a customer service training program, one must consider their effectiveness in light of the survey results. Key questions to consider when judging existing customer service training programs include the following:

- How are we currently training employees to demonstrate compassion, friendliness, and genuine interest in patient well-being?
- What hiring practices target candidates with the most desirable traits?
- How are middle managers in health care settings coaching and rewarding desirable customer service behaviors?
- How is our organization measuring and managing the correlation between employee attitude and patient and physician satisfaction?

Managed care has grown by leaps and bounds since the early '90s and is projected to continue to grow well into the new millennium. As employers drive more and more employees into managed care arrangements, patient satisfaction becomes pivotal in big business decisions.

There is no doubt that a fundamental change is on the horizon. But not everyone in the health care industry is quick to embrace the inevitable increase in customer service demands. Physicians in particular have been lauded for skills and competencies completely unrelated to the human element of medicine. Most physicians were trained to diagnose and treat disease, and they pride themselves on delivering high-quality care measured by cure rates and utilization. Whether or not their patients find them friendly, informative, and genuinely concerned about them as individuals has been traditionally viewed as incidental.

A Look at Revenue Loss

In health care, as with any other business, there are important moments of truth—those crucial points when someone coming into contact with our organization uses that experience to judge its quality. In the course of my career, I have encountered numerous situations in which health care providers have completely blown those crucial moments of truth. Rather than impressing patients and their families, they have alienated them, causing a lifelong loss of revenue for the organization.

Consider the 27-year-old woman whose son was seen by her family's primary care physician. She complained that both the physician and his staff had been rude and discounted her concerns for her sick child. When I approached the physician about the complaint, he responded tersely, "There are plenty of other doctors around. Maybe she'd be happier elsewhere." Having been born and bred in the era of fee-for-service health care, this physician hadn't yet internalized the impact his behavior can have on his reputation, satisfaction ratings, and, hence, his income. But even more damaging is that his reputation is intertwined with that of our community hospital. Area residents see us as one and the same even though the vast majority of the medical staff operate as separate business entities.

When this patient decided to take her son to a neighboring community for care, we all lost. She had to travel out of town when it would have been more convenient for her to drive the six blocks to her former clinic. The physician and the local hospital were losing not just one office visit but possibly a 50-year relationship with a customer who is also the primary decision maker about health care services for herself, her husband, and her three children. Some simple calculations can place a conservative dollar value on this loss. Based on managed care estimates of three office visits per year per covered life at $75 per visit, the loss could be calculated as follows:

Female (27 years old, average life expectancy 77)
50 years × 3 office visits (@$75/visit) = $11,250

Male (27 years old, average life expectancy 75)
48 years × 3 office visits = $10,800

Child (newborn)
77 years × 3 office visits = $17,325

Child (2 years old)
75 years × 3 office visits = $16,875

Child (5 years old)
70 years × 3 office visits = $15,750

Total $72,000

Multiply this figure by the inflationary rate and add the charges for two to three emergency visits and two minor surgeries apiece for a conservative view of the direct financial loss suffered when a medical practice loses one customer. The indirect costs are even more profound. Research confirms that dissatisfied customers tell about 13 other people. If this dissatisfied woman influences 13 other people, the loss will not only be a financial one but a loss of reputation as well.

What Reputation Can Do

The word *reputation* is freely used when discussing public perception. For the hard-core statisticians, the word is too soft to hold any real clout. But for those of us who work in marketing and public relations, reputation is not taken lightly. We understand that reputation is a driving force in consumer decisions. It is what leads a new customer to you or away from you. The origin of the word *reputation* gives credence to the marketers' viewpoint. It is defined as "the general estimation in which a person or thing is held by the public."[4] Its origin is the Latin word *reputatio,* which means a reckoning or the act of counting or computation.

While the definition of the word *reputation* in modern vernacular reinforces the soft image, its origin points back to the link between image and its quantifiable impact. Reputation can be measured by public opinion and quantified further by market share and loyalty. Customers can and will vote with their feet, and often the only deciding factor is reputation. A health care organization can change its reputation only by refilling the communication channels with tales of legendary service. Furthermore, it is only when the individual employee believes and acts on behalf of the organization in every encounter with every customer that the organization will be able to recraft its reputation to one of service excellence.

Don't Just Satisfy Them, Get Them Talking!

When was the last time you made a conscious decision to choose an average product or service? Probably never. Most of us want high-quality, value-added goods and services. Knowing that expectations are higher in health care than in other businesses, it only makes sense to strive for excellence rather than simply hoping not to offend the customer.

Satisfaction or Excellence?

For years, health care providers would conduct patient satisfaction surveys and present the data in terms of averages. However, communicating specific goals that raise the bar for every staff member will bring your organization one step away from average and closer to excellence. Stating your goal specifically will head your team toward the right goalpost. For instance, stating your goal as "95 percent of our patients will rate us excellent or 5 on a 5-point scale" makes the goal clear and understandable.

In his book *Healthcare Marketing in Transition,* Terrence Rynne succinctly defines the various levels of marketing achievement. Rynne uses the ladder of marketing achievement (figure 1-1) to demonstrate that positive word of mouth is the best indicator of high customer satisfaction. Rynne defines name recognition as the lowest rung of the ladder, followed by top-of-mind awareness, preference, use, and reuse.[5]

e 1-1. Ladder of Marketing Achievement

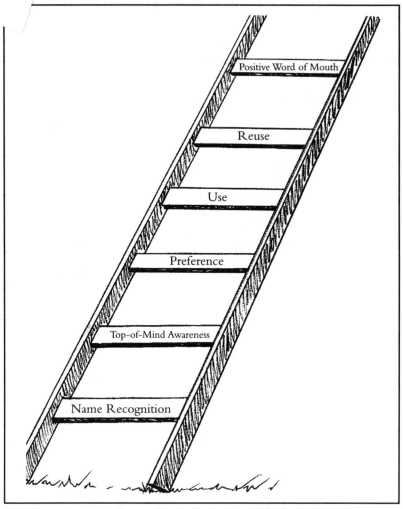

Source: Terrence Rynne, *Healthcare Marketing in Transition* (New York: The McGraw-Hill Companies, Inc., 1997), p. 221.

I use Rynne's ladder during new-employee orientation to demonstrate that advertising and promotion can make an impact on the first three rungs of the ladder, but once customers use our service, the moments of truth they experience will determine the top two rungs. Will they reuse our services? And will they speak highly of their experiences with us? Using Rynne's model, it is easy to demonstrate how every employee plays a crucial role in creating the positive experiences that will lead to reuse and positive word of mouth. Not only do new employees benefit from this visual example of how customer service fits into the organization's marketing achievement, but senior leaders, managers, and long-term employees benefit as well.

In situations where a hospital's or clinic's reputation has been tainted through a history of bad experiences, it becomes a matter of refilling the information channels. The dictionary defines *legend* as: "1. An unverified popular story handed down from earlier times, or 2. A body or collection of such stories that are told over and over."[6] Reputations are built on stories or legends told by patients, their friends, and family members. New employees should be challenged to recognize each encounter as an opportunity to create new legends that will fill the information channels and reroute the rumor mills.

What Would You Like Them to Say about You?

This question, while simple, is one over which each employee can have some influence. Sharing real-life stories with our new hires is one way to bring this point to life. Storytelling provides an opportunity to spotlight the most desirable, patient-focused behaviors performed by everyday people or to give a harsh reminder of the importance of patient perceptions. Here is one story I have shared regularly with new staff.

Recently a friend of mine was hospitalized for the removal of a lump in her breast. Like many women, the time between Sue's positive mammogram and the surgery was filled with tension. At this stage, the nagging concern over the unknown was very troubling.

Sue's deep spirituality gave her a sense of hope, and her long-term relationship with her physician gave her a strong dose of confidence. But in spite of these things, Sue awoke from surgery with a natural level of fear for a woman who had just undergone a lumpectomy. Several unanswered questions nagged at her. What would the biopsy show? What will all of this mean for me? Is my life really about to change?

Waiting for a diagnosis after the surgery was difficult because when Sue awoke from the anesthesia, no one spoke to her. The enormous bandages on her chest revealed little about the surgery's outcome. She had no idea if her breast had been removed or if the surgeon had opted for a simple lumpectomy. Her physical pain further exaggerated her mental anguish. After three unanswered calls to the nurses for pain medication, Sue escalated from annoyed to panic-stricken, then angry. Didn't anyone care? Do they even know I'm here? Maybe no one knows I'm back from surgery. After the fourth call, someone (without introducing herself) promised that she'd get something soon. An hour later, Sue received her first pain medication but not before she got the diagnosis.

She had cancer. The word surged through her like an electrical current. Not since she was a child brushing up against an electric fence on her uncle's farm had Sue felt such a shock. "It's an aggressive type," a whispered voice in the hall said. "No, we're not sure yet if its spread to the lymph nodes or not. She has five daughters; they're sure going to have to be really watchful for the rest of their lives."

"My god," Sue thought, "they're talking about me!" She had been betrayed. Not only did she have to deal with the trauma of cancer, but now Sue had to learn of her diagnosis by overhearing two staff members chatting outside her door.

Sue's story carries with it many lessons for health care workers. There is never, under any circumstances, an excuse for idle chatter about confidential patient matters within earshot of anyone. In this situation, the patient learned of a shocking diagnosis in the most impersonal manner. And had others overheard the information, it could have been a clear breach of confidentiality. Sue was left unattended at a time when she needed information and reassurance as well as pain relief. Even the simplest courtesy of introducing themselves had been overlooked by the staff.

Sue's situation went from bad to worse in terms of customer service. She had just had the worst news of her life and she was in pain, alone, and feeling extremely vulnerable because everyone around her remained anonymous and aloof. "The final straw came when the nurse came in to give me the long-awaited pain medication," Sue explained. "After greeting me with a command to roll over for the shot, the nurse proceeded to try to justify her behavior by explaining that she was having a bad day. Can you imagine? I just looked at her and said, 'You're having a bad day? What about me?' From that point on, all I could think about was getting out of there."

Sue has shared her story with numerous individuals since its occurrence. This particular legend lives on in the small community where she lives and has done much to sway people's opinions of their local hospital.

Although this may have been an isolated incident, it is Sue's personal experience and will hold credibility when she tells it at parties, over bridge games, and at church gatherings. When I share this story with new staff while keeping the name of the organization and patient confidential, the listener is encouraged to relate on an emotional level and, at the same time, consider how the situation could have been different. It provides our new staff members with the opportunity to think about how they would react to a similar situation both from a patient's perspective and from the provider's perspective.

One positive story I like to share with new employees is a prime example of an ordinary person performing an extraordinary act of kindness.

It was late one afternoon and "Phil" was leaving work for the day. A maintenance worker for a large multispecialty clinic, Phil usually had long, physically draining days. On this particular drizzly spring day as Phil drove out of the lot, he noticed a young woman with a baby in her arms and a toddler at her side. The trio stood beside a dilapidated station wagon with a very flat tire. Rather than keep going, Phil stopped to lend a hand. As it turned out, the woman had just been in the urgent care center with her feverish infant. The baby was fussy, the toddler was hungry, and the mother was visibly exhausted. Guessing that the family had limited options, Phil not only offered to change the tire but made a trip to a nearby service station to have the spare filled and the old tire repaired. He had the family wait in his warm car while he made the change and even escorted them home to be sure they arrived safely. Phil could have kept going out of the parking lot that day or settled for calling a tow truck. But Phil is not just a good guy, he's a person who sees himself as a direct extension of his employer—the clinic. When Phil acted, he acted on behalf of his organization and in response to the values he holds dear. He took action to help someone in need and would never have mentioned a word to anyone. But this grateful woman wrote a letter to the administrator praising not only Phil for his kindness but also the clinic for having the good sense to hire wonderful employees like him.

Unfortunately, when I have shared this story with other health care provider groups as an example of service excellence, I've been met with questions such as: "Do you authorize tire changes? What about liability? Isn't that setting a precedent?" These questions are a classic symptom of what is wrong with health care today. We have gone so far in the areas of regulations, policies, and procedures that we have failed to stay in touch with the human elements that attract people into health care professions in the first place. Health care administrators and leaders need to encourage and empower employees to do the right thing at the right time for the right reasons. If we can lead employees with clearly stated values and reward exemplary behaviors, we will surely put the "care" back in health care.

Customer Service as It Relates to Business Development

Say the words *business development* and the first things that come to mind are words like *business plan, line extension, forecasting,* and *market share*. Although all of these elements are important, traditional business development strategies cannot possibly succeed without strong emphasis on customer service. Using Rynne's ladder (figure 1-1), it becomes evident that advertising can take an organization only so far. Then the moments of truth take over. My mother, like many others, always said, "You never get a second chance to make a good first impression." Those first impressions may be formed long before your customers come face-to-face with you. When they call, are they put on hold, transferred to three or four other departments, and made to repeat personal information several times? Can they find your building, office, or suite? Is signage clear? Is parking adequate and convenient? More than once, I have seen patients arrive completely exasperated over confusing instructions, lousy directional signs, and inadequate parking. If the registration clerk hears these tales of woe and simply responds, "Yes I know, you're the fifth one this morning to tell me that," your business plan and marketing plan won't stand much of a chance. But if she addresses their concern with a customer-focused response, the prognosis improves dramatically. For example, imagine the clerk responding to the same scenario described above with: "Thank you so much for telling me this. If you don't mind, I'd like to jot down some more specific information about the difficulties you had and pass them along to our maintenance and plant services department. It is working on new signage and additional parking. Then, I'd also like to make sure your doctor's office staff has a supply of maps so that the doctor's patients won't have trouble finding the hospital from his clinic."

Summary

Moving from name recognition to positive word of mouth requires consistent positive experiences with every encounter between your organization and its customers. But merely understanding this fact and acting on it are two very different things.

This chapter was presented as background information. The remainder of the book is devoted to helping you move beyond understanding and into action directed at achieving a higher level of customer satisfaction throughout your organization.

When it comes to your customers, if you ignore them, they will go away!

References

1. D. Zimmerman, P. Zimmerman, and C. Lund, *The Healthcare Customer Service Revolution: The Growing Impact of Managed Care on Patient Satisfaction* (Chicago: Richard D. Irwin, 1996), p. vii.

2. Dick Davidson, *"Reality Check, Public Perceptions of Health Care and Hospitals,"* report to AHA member CEOs on a nationwide focus group/opinion research survey by the American Hospital Association (1996), p. 6.

3. D. Zimmerman, "Customer Service: The New Battlefield for Market Share," *Healthcare Marketing Abstracts* 12 (1997): 10.

4. *The American Heritage Dictionary of the English Language* (Boston: American Heritage Publishing Co., Inc., 1975), p. 1105.

5. Rynne, Terrence, *Healthcare Marketing in Transition: Practical Answers to Pressing Questions* (Chicago: Richard D. Irwin, 1995), p. 221.

6. *The American Heritage Dictionary of the English Language,* p. 747.

CHAPTER TWO

Setting Your Course— Senior Leadership Takes the Wheel

"Heroic service does not come from policy manuals. It comes from people who care—and from a culture that encourages and models that attitude."
—Valerie Oberle, vice president, Disney University Guest Program[1]

Objectives

After completing this chapter the reader will:

- Be able to articulate the vision and organizational values necessary for customer service excellence

- Identify essential qualities necessary for a strong layer of middle managers

- Be prepared to evaluate middle managers on leadership skills needed for building a customer-focused staff and use the assessment to define training needs

Robert Greenleaf states:

> Caring for persons, the more able and the less able serving each other, is the rock upon which a good society is built. Whereas, until recently, caring was largely person to person, now most of it is mediated through large institutions—often large, complex, powerful, impersonal, not always competent, sometimes corrupt. If a better society is to be built, one that is more just and loving, one that provides greater creative opportunity for its people, then the most open course is to raise both the capacity to serve and the very performance as servant of existing major institutions by new regenerative forces operating within them.[2]

Greenleaf eloquently substantiates the need for leaders to see themselves first as servants to others and then lead from that core philosophy. His thesis extends beyond the CEO to the board of directors or trustees. Greenleaf contends that the trustees' role in appointing the right CEO or administrator to lead the organization is as crucial to organizational personality as it is to the bottom line.

Top-Down Communication

A solid customer service program requires clear expectations and consistent support from the top down and buy-in from the bottom up. It requires setting clear expectations for the management team so that the members understand what is expected of them—not just as employees but also as leaders, role models, disciplinarians, and otherwise shapers of employee behavior. Without a strong foundation built by top leadership, your organization will not achieve a consistent, desirable level of service excellence. As figure 2-1 indicates, clarification and communication of core values by top leadership are the starting points on the road map for success. This chapter directs senior leadership to clarify core values and communicate them clearly to managers and line staff as an essential first step in creating a culture of service excellence. This chapter also helps senior leaders to assess leadership training needs among middle managers.

Figure 2-1. Road Map for Success

Start here.

PHASE 1

(1) Administrative team states vision and support for customer service excellence.

(2) • Clarify vision and core values.
• Identify customer service champion.
• Evaluate middle managers' mind-set and leader qualities.
Identify management training needs.

(3)

(4)

Evaluate Baseline
• Patient satisfaction
• Physician satisfaction
• Employee satisfaction

Form first-generation customer service team.

(5)

Create Standards
• Focus groups
• Review
• Modify

(6)

Training
• Overall objectives
• Identify groups with unique training needs

New Orients
• Expectations

Manager
• Administration expectations
• Coaching
• Monitor/measure

Existing Staff

Complete training corporatewide

(6)

All new hires
Customer service standards in orientation

One Month Later
• Standards
• Assessment of new employees' view of corporate culture

Ongoing Reinforcement

Annual Education Day
• **How can we improve?**

Ongoing training and evaluation for all employees

Performance review
• Evaluate customer service behavior.
• Determine individual training needs.

PHASE 2

Second-generation customer service team focuses on building service-driven departments.

(7)

• Key results area
• Action plans
• Rewards/recognition

Measure results. (10)
• Patient
• Employee
• Medical staff

PHASE 3

Rewards/Recognition for Visionary Leadership

Being Accountable
• To organization
• To administration
• To staff

Supporting Standards
Managing/mentoring and coaching for service excellence

◯ *Denotes related chapter*

19

To say that the administrative team plays a pivotal role in setting the stage for the entire customer service initiative in every organization is a gross understatement. Without leadership that sets the stage and walks the talk, there is little hope for fostering a culture of customer service excellence. In most cases, it is the top leadership that consistently communicates the organization's mission and vision. To spearhead a solid customer service initiative, the CEO and senior leaders must be involved. I strongly recommend that, at a minimum, senior leaders read the first three chapters of this book, then convene for a discussion of its contents.

Managers, on the other hand, must understand the importance of customer service in the hiring and review process as well as in day-to-day supervision and role modeling. They must continually uphold and communicate the mission and vision to their departments. Long-term employees may have fallen into some bad habits that were either tolerated or ignored because no one really clarified the organization's expectations. Newly hired employees need guidance about expectations and corporate culture. They too are new customers and are forming opinions, not only about their new role, but also about the entire organization. It is up to administration or senior leadership to set the course of action by stating the core values that drive the organization.

Articulating Core Values

An administrator hoping to improve customer service in his or her organization must first take an honest look at the organization's core values, not only as a leader and shaper of the work environment, but also as a person. This is essential because in order to lead others, you must have a sense of self. This sense will shape your thoughts and actions that, in turn, drive your behavior. And like it or not, your behavior is what the managers and employees see and believe.

When your staff see you as passionate about quality and commitment to patient care and customer service, they will be much more likely to follow in your footsteps. When they see you as blasé, they are equally likely to follow your lead. To get at some of your personal core values, ask yourself the following questions:

- What do I believe that we, as health care providers, can contribute to the community? To the individual?
- What is unique about health care compared with other service industries?
- How do I measure my worth to the organization? Is it strictly in terms of financial success or am I invested in building stronger leaders? Is my worth gauged according to patient and customer satisfaction?
- How do I want our organization to be viewed by the community?
- How do I want to be viewed by the employees?

Answers to these questions provide a clearer view of your values in relation to your role as a senior leader. Once these are clear to you, you will be able to ask yourself some additional questions directed at how well you communicate these values and model behaviors consistent with these values.

John Kosanovich, CEO of Watertown Area Health Services, where I work, uses a simple phrase to share his values with employees throughout the organization. Beginning on the first day of employment and continuing through written and verbal messages, John tells the staff to screen their actions with the following statement: "We want Watertown Area Health Services to be a place where patients choose to come for care, where physicians want to practice, and where employees want to work." He stresses that by using this as a screening device for all actions and communications, each of us will be making the organization a better place.

Probably the most crucial role of the administrator or senior leader is the ability and desire to build a strong layer of middle managers. It is also the most time consuming and difficult. Most of us don't have the chance to start with a clean slate and fill positions with our handpicked candidates. Instead, we passively acquire what is already in place and deal with it in a number of ways. Wiping out the existing middle layer is seldom an option for a new CEO. In doing so, he or she would be creating fear and dissension throughout the organization. Conversely, if the CEO retains middle managers who do not behave consistently with the stated core values, the administrator creates confusion and distrust at all levels. The middle road is to work diligently at building up the strength and quality of the middle managers.

Clarifying expectations of managers and then holding them accountable are absolutely essential. White and Lee state, "The president who thinks he or she can delegate the job of quality service management to others is going to see it slip through the cracks. Like everyone else, managers do what the president inspects, not what he expects. Only where the CEO requires regular reports and gets personally involved in hearing complaints, solving problems, creating incentives, giving rewards and role modeling will the effort be more than superficially successful."[3]

Articulating Organizational Values

Once you have clarified your own values, you can shift your focus to those of the organization. Does the organization have clear values? What are they and how are they communicated? If the values have never been clearly articulated, here's your chance to start anew. Values are typically the foundation on which the mission statement is based.

Begin with the mission statement. Although you know it will be neither profound nor original, pull it out, dust it off, and take a good look at the words that are supposed to be the driving force behind your organization's culture. Pick out some key words that form the core of the message. Very often these words will include *service, healing, care, excellence,* and *compassion.* If you continue examining these key words, many of them will lead you right into customer service behaviors.

If historical archives from your hospital cannot provide you with original value statements, you may have to craft them based on what you know and believe. The key is to keep them closely linked to the mission and vision, simple, and memorable.

If core values have never been clarified and communicated, you will have to lead the process. This is a crucial step in the customer service process. You may want to use focus groups to steer the development (see chapter 5).

Holy Cross Hospital in Chicago has a set of core values that is clear, memorable, and evident throughout the organization. CEO Mark Clement makes certain that the values are clearly articulated and interwoven into the actions of every employee (partner) within the organization, and in the mid-1990s he used these values to lead the hospital through a financial and service turnaround. The values are service, excellence, respect, value, and enthusiasm (SERVE).[4]

What Message Have You Given Managers?

Chances are good that if you had to struggle to identify or define core values, you have never really articulated them clearly to the management team, nor have you tied them to leadership performance expectations. Without this step, you have sent your managers on a trip without a clear destination, timeline, or road map. The bad news is that in the meantime they have been leading the troops. But where? The good news, however, is that it's not too late. Time spent on clarifying core values for the organization is time well spent.

Once you have articulated the organization's core values, consider how well your middle managers are currently supporting those values. They may have already been doing a good job if the culture has been established with a customer-focused philosophy. If they are not, ask yourself:

• Have I clarified these values and held managers accountable for demonstrating and leading others in a manner consistent with these values?

- What additional tools might the managers need to feel successful as leaders or role models in the area of customer service? Do they need more training?
- What is the culture that the managers currently foster among others?
- Am I stating my expectations clearly enough?
- Am I recognizing and reinforcing desirable leadership qualities among middle managers?

At this point, it may be beneficial to conduct a leadership skills assessment of the middle managers in your organization. By establishing a baseline of skills you will be able to tailor training efforts needed for future progress. An outside consultant may be useful for this task because he or she can bring a degree of anonymity and objectivity to the assessment.

Leadership Skills Assessment

Fostering leadership skills among middle management and supervisors is not so much rocket science as it is a long-term commitment. Senior leadership cannot expect middle management to perform to a certain level of expectations unless, first, they clearly understand the expectations and, second, they have the skills needed to succeed.

Spelling out specific expectations and establishing a method to measure leadership performance against those expectations is the first step. You cannot "grade" management arbitrarily and expect to maintain any credibility.

Until 1998, my organization, Watertown Memorial Hospital in Wisconsin, was using the same tool to measure leadership performance for all employees. Managers were evaluated on the same criteria as housekeepers, nurses, and food service workers. Taking a new look at how we measured managers' performance was imperative to our cultural shift. For example, the evaluation described individuals' customer service behavior, but not whether they fostered positive behavior in others.

Although this measure may be appropriate for the average employee, it isn't what is most important in assessing the middle manager's leadership skills.

Working with a team of middle managers and an outside facilitator, we crafted an evaluation tool that now brings managers much closer to the hospital's corporate goals. Some of the skills measured include the following:

- Creating and communicating the customer service vision and strategy
- Promoting and supporting customer service
- Encouraging employee involvement and empowerment
- Coaching and reinforcing performance
- Building teamwork
- Developing self and others
- Creating a climate of open communication
- Decision-making/analytical skills
- Interpersonal skills
- Organizational skills

Along with proper training, accountability is a key factor in leadership development. Baptist Hospital CEO Quint Studer links his hospital's turnaround to a shift in managers' accountability. Studer states, "All our leaders get report cards every 90 days. That's how we align behaviors to our goals and how we can reward objectively." Baptist Hospital managers are graded in four categories: customer service, which is gauged according to the hospital's position in a national benchmark; efficiency; expense management; and staff turnover.[5]

Do You Have the Right People in Management?

For decades, health care has rewarded managers based on one thing—the bottom line. If she stayed within the budget and ran a tight ship, she was a good manager. That's not enough in today's competitive environment. A strong organization requires strong middle management.

One of the toughest tasks for senior leadership is having to ask a manager to leave. But after you have clarified expectations for your managers, held them accountable, trained, mentored, cajoled, and threatened, it's time to take action. Keeping a middle manager in place who clearly does not fit with your message erodes your credibility as a leader.

Leading toward a Corporate Culture of Service Excellence

Interviews with consultants and CEOs have helped to shape this chapter. All were chosen based on their perception of where their institutions are in relation to the customer service challenge. Some are just beginning, some are still struggling, and others are long on their way to demonstrating significant success in customer service. From these experiences with senior leaders I have come to one conclusion: If you are not personally very clear about the core values of your organization, you are not yet prepared to lead others toward a corporate culture of service excellence. If you cannot spend the time, energy, and resources needed to build a strong middle management, stop here. Nothing else you do in the area of fostering a customer-oriented environment will matter. If you cannot place trust in, and empower, every employee in your organization to take some risk, the rest of this book was written for someone else.

Albert Schweitzer said, "Example is not the main thing in influencing others. It is the only thing." Asking your public relations staff or human resources staff to "train" for customer service without clarity of corporate values and mission is like sending your organization on a trip without a destination, road map, money, or timeline and then telling them to hurry up and get there.

Now pull out the strategic plan. If your organization is like everyone else's in health care, the ink isn't dry before you have to draft the next one. But look at it anyway. Now compare it to the mission. Is there some disparity? Is there anything of substance in the strategic plan that could help you to achieve your mission? I hope you will find many common denominators. Now the challenge is making sure that you link the vision and mission to performance expectations.

At Watertown Memorial Hospital, as at many other hospitals, the leadership shared a clear vision of what constituted good customer service. The problem, however, was our own expectations. We began with the assumption that everyone else in the organization was comfortable with a commonsense approach to customer service. In other words, "Do the right thing for the right reasons." But decades of a policy-driven culture had framed staff dependency on black and white rules that left little, if any, latitude for independent thinking and problem solving. We were a commonsense leadership team leading people who were waiting to be told what to do next.

One of our greatest challenges was to foster a culture shift that set clear expectations for service excellence yet empowered and rewarded critical thinking and independent problem solving. After 30 years with the same administrator at the helm, many employees had come to rely on the security of staying within their own department or silo and not having to think about taking responsibility for anything that was not stated in their job description. Performance reviews were generic and kept separate from pay increases. Years of across-the-board raises left many employees comfortable with the status quo. When an attitude of "we've always done it this way" is rewarded with pay increases and job security, it's a little difficult to create a desire for change.

Making Sure All the Leadership Team Are on the Same Page

Assuming that all of the leadership team are thinking and expecting the same things with regard to customer service can be a critical error. Begin by having an open discussion about the vision for customer service and back into the specifics of what is required for each person involved in shaping the culture.

Call the top administrative team together for an open dialogue about core values and how they relate to patient satisfaction and the customer service initiative. Keep in mind that knowing the importance of good customer service and leading an organization toward service excellence are not one and the same. Solid leadership requires defining the vision, then coaching, training, and navigating the organization toward that vision. In almost every organization, the CEO cannot be expected to be the one to train, supervise, and reward positive customer service behaviors. He or she can, however, value customer service enough to support an ongoing initiative, model desirable behaviors, and hold management accountable for setting and achieving customer service goals.

If there has never been a formal customer service program initiated within your organization, an outside consultant may be an asset at this point. A consultant with expertise in leadership training and customer service could lead the administrative team in discussions that can set the stage for the corporatewide initiative, or you can create a homegrown program with the assistance of this book.

Key discussion points to cover with the administrative team include the following:

- Why customer service? (See chapter 1.) Present a clear overview of the financial and market share value of a solid customer service initiative.
- How do we know where we are today? If it is available, present baseline customer satisfaction data, which may include employee satisfaction, patient satisfaction, and physician satisfaction data. If unavailable, stress the need to create the baseline data (see chapter 4).
- What are our core values? How do we communicate them? How do we tie them to performance reviews, rewards, and recognition?

- Are there systems in place that support management efforts to guide employee behavior (for example, disciplinary action policy, merit rewards, and pay for performance)?

In order to get a broader view of common CEO perspectives beyond my own experience, I sought input from other professionals with expertise in customer service development. Marsha Borling, owner of Borling and Associates in Gurnee, Illinois, specializes in customer service development, executive team development, and strategic planning. Borling states:

> One thing that keeps many top executives from embracing customer service improvement is a simple matter of priorities. Some have a singular focus—the bottom line. They view customer service as "fluff"—and it shows. Without always realizing it, that's the message they send throughout the organization. A culture shift toward improved customer service has a slow, steady impact on the bottom line. That can be a hard sell for executives who are looking for a quick hit to the bottom line, such as the hit that strategies like reengineering can bring. Building buy-in at the top can be a difficult challenge, but without it, you cannot possibly create an environment of customer service excellence.

Borling makes a strong case for the link between employee morale and patient satisfaction. She stresses the importance of helping leadership to understand this link and gain concrete baseline data that will quantify employee morale. As with any important change, it is essential to understand where you are today in order to set specific goals and a road map for getting there. She states:

> Begin with measurement. You need to know the current level of employee morale. Find a consulting firm with the ability to compare you to others in the industry on some issues that are inherent to health care. It is also important to identify and understand the correlating factors that drive your employees' job satisfaction up or down. Interviews, focus groups, and exit interviews can all help to identify these drivers. Together, this

information will paint a picture of what needs to be addressed. With an adequate assessment, specific strategies and tactics will be more effective.

Once you have the willingness and interest of the leadership, it's time to look at one of the most pivotal elements that are shaping the personality of your organization every day, in every corner—the management. Some key questions for the top leadership include the following:

- Are we building a stronger layer of middle managers?
- Have we made our expectations clear to managers?
- Have we developed tools to measure and reinforce positive management performance?
- Are we holding managers accountable for monitoring and measuring staff performance?
- Have we provided them with the tools that they need to grow in their role as managers?

I contend that you can teach anyone to monitor time cards, schedule shifts, or balance a budget, but it takes an unusual individual to encourage people to grow. Today's ideal managers should more accurately be called coaches, role models, or mentors. When hiring middle managers, it's important for the leadership to have a clear vision of what is most important to the organization. Years ago, it may have been more appropriate to hire individuals who could maintain tight reins over a group of subordinates. Today, however, with the rapid speed of change in health care, middle management must be multifaceted with exceptional people skills. Furthermore, leadership development is paramount to an organization's success. Administration loses credibility if we ask managers to change, then don't provide them with the tools to make change happen.

Today's Health Care Managers

Fostering a culture of customer service requires that managers not only buy into the vision on a personal level but also put it into action every day. This mind-set is not an easy one to achieve. After all, aren't we looking for clinical expertise? It has taken health care decades to evolve to the point of valuing management skills as unique and desirable traits beyond clinical expertise. Historically, the best clinicians were made nurse managers. Never mind that they had no management skills; they could learn. Or could they?

A classmate of mine in graduate school had made the transition from clinician to manager to customer service trainer for his large integrated delivery system. "Steven" states, "I used to hire respiratory therapists that were up on the latest treatment modalities. I wanted to be sure they knew how to use the technology. I sincerely never screened them for desirable behaviors outside their clinical prowess. Today, I have a totally different mind-set. If they have the degree and the personality and the desire, I can teach them to push the right buttons at the right time. I can't order them to have a better disposition."

In stark contrast to Steven's viewpoint, a long-time manager of a nursing unit brought out the more common sentiments of managers. When "Mary" was confronted with information about the abrupt behavior and rude remarks to coworkers and patients of one of her staff nurses, Mary felt reluctant to press the issue to the point of dismissal, even after several formal reprimands. "But she's such a good nurse," Mary explained. The challenge was evident. She had to get clear on what characteristics make a good nurse. In addition to the proper licensure and clinical competencies, Mary needed to define the other qualities that are needed to be a "good" nurse in our organization.

If being a good nurse meant starting an IV on the first try, or interpreting EKGs like a pro, this nurse had it all. But if it meant doing all those things plus demonstrating compassion, care, respect, and consideration for all those with whom she came in contact, she was clearly not qualified for her position. Rewarding and recognizing desirable traits in staff requires that we get clear on the values.

All employers can apply this concept to the hiring process, as emphasized in the Covey bestseller *Seven Habits of Highly*

Successful People.[6] When we become involved in the hiring process, we need to have a clear idea of the desirable qualities that we are seeking for the position and use questions that will unveil these qualities when we interview.

Holy Cross Hospital in Chicago has been lauded nationally for its ability to turn patient satisfaction around in a short time. Holy Cross now requires everyone applying for a position with the organization to view a 20-minute video about its corporate values; it then asks them how they feel they would fit into the organization in light of these values. The hospital also uses a team interview approach that identifies a candidate's ability to work with others.[7]

Mentor, Monitor, and Measure

Managers, like administrators, must walk the talk of customer service. If the employees don't see the manager as a team player and one who consistently treats others with respect and dignity, the battle is lost. Mentoring requires ongoing role modeling as well as reinforcing positive behavior. Managers who don't take the time to monitor employee behavior will miss opportunities to redirect undesirable behavior as well as commend desirable conduct.

CEO Quint Studer spoke with me about his expectations for managers in monitoring and reinforcing customer service behaviors among his staff. Baptist Hospital employees are expected to introduce themselves to patients consistently and provide patients with clear information about their care plan for the day. In order to make sure that happens, managers get involved. The goal is not to spy on employees but to seize opportunities to reinforce positive behaviors. In Studer's words:

> I expect nurse managers to make rounds and visit with every patient on their units daily. During that visit, the manager introduces herself, asks the patient who is their care provider today, and asks if they know what is planned for their care today. This simple action creates an opportunity to give the

staff nurse immediate feedback related to our goals. For example, the nurse manager can now approach the staff nurse and say, "Cheryl, I just wanted to let you know how pleased I am to see that every one of your patients is clear about today's treatment plan. It's obvious that you took time to not only introduce yourself but to review today's plans. Thanks for keeping our goals in mind."

Evaluating employees on customer service skills will be easier once the organization defines its standards (see chapter 5). But far more important than the annual review is the daily observation of, reinforcement from, and role modeling by managers. These functions are time consuming, but you must demonstrate that you value the effort enough to put your time and energy into it.

Training objectives for managers are strikingly different from those for the line staff and will be outlined in chapter 6. Although all employees must understand and adhere to customer service standards, it is the managers who must hire for, measure, and monitor these qualities among their staff. And in order to be effective, managers will need to know what is expected of them and what support can be expected from the administrative team.

Very early on in the customer service initiative, administration should outline and communicate expectations for the managers in terms of their roles. At the same time, the managers will need the reassurance that administration will help them in fostering the leadership skills required. These often include coaching, conflict resolution, handling confrontation, hiring practices, and measuring and managing staff behavior. One of the simplest, but core, training needs is a review of evaluation tools and disciplinary policies and procedures.

Clarify What Is Expected of Managers

Each manager must understand that he or she is accountable to the organization for customer satisfaction. If administration plans to hold managers accountable, it will need a means for measuring baseline customer satisfaction and ongoing improvement. Satisfaction measurement must be consistent and reliable in order to gain credibility with the managers and employees. By providing each department with patient satisfaction data on a regular basis, administration will be able to set specific and realistic goals for service improvement. Measures for customer satisfaction by which managers can be evaluated include patient satisfaction and employee satisfaction (including turnover).

One interviewed CEO stated that managers in his system are held accountable in four key results areas and are evaluated quarterly. These areas are patient satisfaction, employee turnover, quality improvement initiatives, and fiscal responsibility. He emphasized that holding the managers accountable in this manner is very labor intensive but had brought about excellent results. Not only did his organization improve patient satisfaction scores, decrease turnover, and attain a healthier bottom line, but the managers felt a greater sense of pride and accomplishment knowing that they were in sync with the strategic objectives of the organization.

Bottom-Line Results

Gaining buy-in to customer service can be challenging if managers have not been held accountable for satisfaction in the past. Holding managers accountable for unit-specific satisfaction results is essential but often a hard sell. In speaking with other health care leaders, I have found that staff and managers have challenged them on the use of patient satisfaction data. All of us hear a similar litany of excuses, including, but not limited to, the following:

- "Our patients are sicker, so of course our scores would be lower."
- "We have the most patients, so of course our scores would be lower."

- "Look, we're busy saving lives and can't focus on courtesy. Of course our scores would be lower."

There are often a million and one excuses about why satisfaction is low. Allowing managers to explain away poor results won't improve your organization's status. It is important to lead the effort with high-quality, consistent, and reliable data (see chapter 5) and let managers know what is expected of them. For example, you may want to tell them, "You are personally accountable for your unit scores. I expect you to share the good and bad news with your staff consistently and involve them in action plans to address problems. I also expect you to involve staff in rewards and recognition for improvement."

Speak to the managers in terms that they will understand. Not everyone in health care is a statistician, but everyone is familiar with a common set of baseline numbers known as vital signs. Use this analogy for explaining the need for satisfaction data. Clinical professionals can easily equate patient satisfaction measures with vital signs. When a patient presents in the emergency room, delivery room, or clinic office, the first assessments are the patient's blood pressure, pulse, temperature, and respiration. These vital signs provide crucial information about the patient's current condition, and they are compared against universal benchmarks of 120/80, 64, 98.6, and 18, respectively. Just as a physician wouldn't attempt to make an accurate diagnosis without a thorough assessment, health care professionals cannot make necessary improvements if they don't know how they are doing in the first place.

Reinforcing Positive Behavior

Many of us were raised with the belief that complimenting people will make them cocky or conceited. All too often, managers refrain from giving a compliment because they feel it isn't necessary. As part of leadership training, managers will benefit from sessions on coaching and feedback for guiding performance to match organizational expectations.

When discussing the issue of reinforcing positive behavior with a group of managers, one 30-year veteran in nursing management stated, "That's their job. I shouldn't have to be following people around all day applauding them for something they should be doing anyway." It didn't take long for the consequences of her attitude to surface as a link between high staff turnover and low patient satisfaction.

Reinforcing positive behavior isn't a simple matter of following people around saying "atta boy" and patting them on the back all day. It's making an effort to show that you notice and appreciate each employee for his or her unique style. After all, it is employees' interactions with patients and coworkers thousands of times a week that will make the difference between patient loyalty or attrition.

Quint Studer says, "We throw compliments around like manhole covers." Managers will make the most headway with their employees by getting back to some of the most basic principles. Saying "thank you" doesn't cost the organization a dime but will let the recipients know that their efforts and contributions are appreciated. Senior leaders can help to reinforce this by setting a good example. Managers, too, like their department staff, need feedback to reinforce positive behavior. Senior leaders (the CEO and administrative team) need to acknowledge good coaching and leadership skills among the managers on a regular basis.

Eliminating Problem Behavior

Just as you want managers to reinforce the positive behavior of their staff, they also need to be accountable for eliminating negative behavior. After working with a group at Watertown Memorial Hospital to develop customer service standards, I asked the focus group participants to give me feedback on whether they felt the standards were achievable in our organization. There was clearly a high degree of skepticism. Delving further, I found that there were some long-term "bad apples"—employees with a history of nearly 20 years of patient and coworker complaints about bad attitudes and rude behavior. Their managers had not acted on the behavior and, in turn, the administration had not acted to correct the manager's negligence. I was told very bluntly that there was little, if any, faith that the bad apples would be weeded out.

My initial shock and discouragement led to an action plan. Listening to the focus groups made it clear that there was a trickle-down effect that had to be changed. Somehow, complacency among the leadership had spread like a virus, threatening the health of the customer service initiative. We needed a clear message from the top down that customer service is, and will continue to be, a crucial element of our business. This message was communicated in the management customer service training session but required repetition for months to come.

Building a stronger layer of middle managers is crucial to the success of any organization, but particularly those committed to customer service excellence. To do the subject justice is beyond the scope of this work. The most important consideration at this point is to recognize the unique needs of the management layer in terms of its training needs and administration's responsibility for holding managers accountable. Customer service training objectives are more clearly outlined in chapter 6.

It's Not a Program—It's a Way of Life

All too often employees are presented with a special training program that is here today and gone tomorrow. Two or three hours of customer service training with an outside authority will not bring about lasting change. In order to weave a customer service philosophy throughout the fabric of your organization, there must be commitment to making it more than a training program. It must be viewed as a way of life. Beginning with the administration's vision and values and continuing through management's daily coaching and reinforcement, customer service excellence requires heightened awareness and ongoing effort. Administration has to set the stage for the rest of the employees and managers. Believing in the value of customer service and acting out a specific role are two very different issues. Management must be accountable for reinforcing positive behavior, eliminating negative behavior, and developing leadership skills that will help to build top performers. Similarly, each individual must operate, not from policies about customer service, but from the vision and core values that form the basis for the corporate culture.

Summary

An administration that can clearly define and communicate core values has taken an essential first step in creating a culture of service excellence. But to be most effective, a customer service–driven organization must see and respect the different needs and duties of each of its various constituents. While everyone is accountable for his or her own behavior, managers and administrators are accountable for guiding performance to match organizational values, goals, and expectations. Leadership behavior is learned. An ongoing program of leadership training must run parallel to the customer service training in order to ensure success (see figure 2-1). By investing time and energy in leadership development, you will be setting the course for a successful customer service initiative.

After clarifying core values, the next challenge is creating a method for clearly and consistently disseminating them throughout the organization. Once the administrative team has defined the values and determined its commitment to customer service and leadership development, it's time to appoint a customer service champion to spearhead the remaining facets. Chapter 3 outlines the process for selecting a champion to lead the initiative.

References

1. Valerie Oberle, vice president, Disney University Guest Program, quoted in *Chicken Soup for the Soul at Work* (Deerfield Beach, FL: Health Communications Inc., 1996), p. 114.

2. Robert Greenleaf, *Servant Leadership, A Journey into the Nature of Legitimate Power and Greatness* (New York: Paulist Press, 1977), p. 49.

3. T. White and F. Lee, "Quality Through Customer Service," *Healthcare Forum Journal* (July/August 1990): 30.

4. "Service Excellence Institute," conference at Holy Cross Hospital (June 8–9, 1998).

5. "The 90-Day Checkup," *INC.* (March 1999), p. 111.

6. Stephen Covey, *Seven Habits of Highly Successful People* (New York: Simon & Schuster, 1989).

7. Vicki Piper, "Building the Right Team," conference presentation, Holy Cross Hospital Service Excellence Institute, Chicago (June 9, 1998).

CHAPTER THREE

Championing Buy-In and Ownership— You Can't Do It Alone

Objectives

After completing this chapter the reader will:

- Understand the need for an internal champion to lead the organization's customer service initiative

- Understand how to gain input from employees at all levels of the organization

- Have the basic criteria for selecting members for the first-generation customer service team

- Have the tools for leading the team in establishing clear goals

A winning team needs a good coach. Imagine football players at the sidelines ready to take the field. Adrenaline pumping, they're fired up and ready to win, but they have no game plan. In fact, they aren't even sure which goal post is theirs. To make matters worse, they don't have a coach.

Embarking on a customer service initiative without a champion is a sure prescription for failure. The champion takes the role of the head coach in sizing up the turf, assessing the opponents, and exploiting the team's greatest strengths. Although the initiative requires unwavering commitment from the CEO, it is not very likely that the CEO will be able to serve as the customer service champion. In most cases, the service champion will be at the CEO's right hand, helping to relay his or her message and keeping the initiative in motion.

In chapter 2 we identified the importance of top leadership's commitment to customer service. The remainder of this book will operate with the assumption that the CEO and top leadership are in full support of the initiative and hold it as a core strategy and objective for the organization's success.

The Customer Service Champion

As mentioned earlier in this book, a successful initiative will require perseverance and vision. The personal qualities of the customer service champion are as important as the tools and tactics. Think of yourselves as building a landmark monument. Of course you will need an array of tools, but without a visionary design and the skill of a talented carpenter, you will never complete the task. Your customer service champion must be the architect and carpenter needed to structure the customer service initiative.

When searching for the ideal person within your organization to spearhead the customer service initiative, consider personal qualities and look beyond titles. To be successful, the service champion must be a leader in the truest sense of the word. He or she must be persuasive, persistent, organized, a visionary, and well respected by the employees and top leadership within the organization. Enthusiasm is another essential quality. A person who is passionate about the importance of customer service excellence will make far more progress than one who has only a cerebral connection to the subject. Metaphorically speaking, enthusiasm is the quality that connects the brain with the heart. And, finally, the ideal individual will be an excellent communicator capable of persuasive public address as well as one-on-one coaching.

The customer service champion will get farther faster if he or she is in a position of authority. Again, this authority doesn't necessarily mean the title; it simply means that the champion would have the ear and full support of the CEO and key decision makers. In order to get things done, the customer service champion must have the authority to cut through bureaucratic red tape and perhaps shake up a few old policies that have prevented individuals from making the best decisions for their customers. The customer service champion must also be a skilled facilitator who can guide groups of individuals from brainstorming and idea development to specific action plans. Ideally, you will find this customer service champion at the senior leader level.

If you are fortunate enough to have several qualified candidates, you may need more information to coax the cream to the top. Ask the candidates the following questions:

- Where do you see our organization in five years in terms of customer service?
- If you were in charge of a corporatewide customer service initiative, where would you begin?
- Who else would you involve to help you reach your goals?
- How does customer service mesh with the organization's mission?

In considering the responses, it's best to look for answers that indicate the desire for a grassroots approach rather than a mandate from above. Individuals who see the value of building buy-in from all levels will be more successful than the person who talks only about policies.

It's improbable that most organizations will identify a candidate whose sole function will be that of the customer service initiative. In fact, I strongly recommend that the customer service champion have other visible responsibilities because he or she needs to demonstrate that customer service behavior is not an add-on for anyone. Customer service behavior is simply a part of any position within the organization. By having other responsibilities, the customer service champion will stay connected to more people at various levels.

The characteristics of the customer service champion are a predictor of the overall success of the initiative. In summary, these include the following qualities:

- *Leadership ability.* The customer service champion will need to guide others in setting and achieving goals.
- *Persuasiveness.* The customer service champion must have the ability to influence others to examine their own behavior and act according to stated values. A convincing individual will motivate others to action.
- *Facilitating skills.* The champion will need to guide the team's creative energy into achievable goals.
- *Persistence.* The task at hand will require repetition and reminders. The customer service champion will have to continually bring the messages back to administration from the organization and vice versa. The service champion must help administrators understand their role in the training and leadership of employees. This quality will prevent the initiative from crashing and burning.
- *Organizational skills.* Juggling priorities and demands is necessary because he or she will be balancing the customer service initiative along with other responsibilities. In addition, as corporate goals are clarified, the customer service champion will need to keep tabs on multiple project teams.

- *Vision.* The customer service champion must be able to see past where the organization is today to where it wishes to be in the future and be able to visualize his or her role in that process.
- *Enthusiasm.* This person must be passionate enough about customer service to keep others excited about their progress.
- *Communication skills.* The customer service champion will need to lead training sessions and team meetings as well as conduct individual coaching discussions. The ability to communicate clearly and with respect is vital to the program's success.
- *Authority.* The customer service champion will likely have to challenge the status quo over and over in the process of altering the existing culture. Being in a position of authority will help others to recognize that it is not only OK to question the status quo; it is encouraged if it will improve service.

Identifying and appointing the customer service champion is the critical first step in creating the first-generation customer service team. The momentum is building at this point in the process and needs to be channeled. By creating the customer service team, the champion will be building collaboration and systemwide buy-in to customer service, which is essential to fostering the grassroots approach.

Creating a Customer Service Team

When a professional sports team drafts players, serious thought is given to the strengths and abilities each individual will bring to the team. If you were to select a basketball team composed of individuals with the same set of skills, they may not have the strength and stamina necessary for a winning season. Instead, you would seek some players for speed and others for height, but all would need shooting prowess and the ability to work with others.

When selecting members for a customer service team, it is important to consider the strengths, skills, and circle of influence each member brings to the table. Ideally you will want to strike a balance between direct care providers and support services, management and line staff, and hospital employees and representatives from affiliated services (clinics, skilled nursing care, home health, assisted living). But be careful not to look at titles alone. Consider the personality and style of each individual on the team. You will need to balance the thinkers and doers with the kind and caring types. All add value to your organization, and all types will bring balance to your team.

Bigger isn't always better when it comes to teams. Any more than ten members and your team could become unmanageable. Any fewer than six and you may not have the mass to create the influence or the manpower needed to complete essential tasks. Creating the right team is essential to your plan for success. Too many members can be as bad as too few.

The charter members of our customer service team at Watertown Area Health Services actually evolved from the core group that had revamped the patient survey methodology and data analysis. Once that task was completed, we shifted our focus to what could be done to improve the findings. Several of our original team members wanted to continue on the new customer service team, but a few others decided to drop out once our original goal (data analysis) had been achieved. Before creating an all-new team, you may want to look over existing teams to determine if customer service would fit well with one of them. If not, the customer service champion will need to build a new team. Following the guidelines in this chapter will help to form a team that is consistent with a grassroots approach.

Once our administrative team had determined the need for improved customer service, we put out a call for team members through the employee newsletter and made announcements at the monthly management education meeting. At first we found ourselves slightly heavy on the management and patient care sides, so we had a second draft that targeted hospitality services (dietary and housekeeping), maintenance, business office, and our satellite community clinics. The customer service champion screened the volunteers through a discussion of customer service philosophies, recommendations from staff who could verify a candidate's ability to influence others, and a candidate's reputation for customer service and task follow-through.

Lessons Learned from Team Member Selection

Our first year at Watertown as a newly formed team was a very productive one with the creation of standards and corporate-wide training sessions. It wasn't until after these initial projects quieted down, however, that we took a fresh look at the composition of our team. We noticed a few gaps that should have been more evident from the beginning. Our hospital, like many, sees the largest number of patients on an outpatient basis. The greatest number of these enter through our urgent care and emergency department. This area is notorious for having the highest number of complaints. We had been remiss not to include a representative from the emergency department who would link the department efforts with the organizationwide initiative.

The volunteers were the second group that had been inadvertently omitted. Although our auxiliary members had been required to attend the customer service training, we had failed to include a representative from the hospital auxiliary on the customer service team. With hundreds of individuals donating thousands of hours to our hospital and affiliated services every year, it was obvious we had missed a golden opportunity. That was soon corrected and now we have at least one delegate from the auxiliary as well as the volunteer coordinator. This link not only gives us insight into a vital group within our organization, but it also provides the team with additional support without using precious staff resources. Keep in mind that over time the composition of the team will (and should) change.

Getting Support from the Top

Each team for the various initiatives in our organization has a sponsor from the administrative team. Although the teams remain fairly autonomous, having an administrative sponsor helps to keep their mission and strategies front and center. It also serves to link other initiatives to individual team efforts and keep the administrative team up-to-date on the various initiatives taking place throughout the system. Having an administrator sponsor can also be valuable in cutting through bureaucratic red tape. In order to challenge the status quo in the name of customer service, the team will need authority early on.

Creating a Team Mission Statement

Once your team is in place, you will need to set a clear direction. To ensure that our team's course was not divergent from the hospital's, we began by reviewing our hospital mission statement. As simplistic and logical as this may seem, I have found it to be a grounding element for each new endeavor undertaken in our organization. It also serves to keep the mission as the focus. By reviewing the hospital mission statement, each of us was starting out at home base and could relate our new efforts to the overriding purpose of the organization as a whole.

The next step for the team is to create a team mission statement. The experts tell us that in order to be effective, a mission statement must be succinct and memorable. The succinct part can be difficult when you gather 10 to 12 creative individuals into a room and say, "Let's write a mission statement." A more direct approach is to lead a group discussion around two to three key questions such as: "What do we hope to achieve?" "Why is customer service important to our organization?" "How does customer service fit with our corporate mission?"

Using a flip chart, overhead transparencies, or newsprint sheets, record participants' remarks and keep them visible throughout the discussion.

When leading a group in mission statement development, I try not to let them spend time on "wordsmithing" the final version. Trying to create exact verbiage with a large group is frequently a fruitless and time-consuming endeavor. Instead, try to concentrate on key phrases or concepts that resurface in the discussion and write these on the chart or newsprint sheets. Verify the core concepts with the group and promise to return with a working draft of a mission statement. This saves time and avoids frustration, particularly if group members are good with ideas and not with the written word. Create the first draft and disseminate it with the meeting minutes with instructions for the members to review it and make their edits prior to the next meeting. Let the group know that the team's goals can be stated separately from the mission statement.

The mission statement formulated at Watertown in 1997 is simple and to the point. It reads: "The mission of the customer service team is to create and foster a sound customer service philosophy and environment throughout Watertown Area Health Services resulting in improved customer satisfaction and loyalty. We define our key customers as patients, physicians, visitors and employees."

There are several books that specifically address the subject of writing a mission statement if you need more help. The main idea is to make sure that the mission statement is succinct, memorable, and tied to the corporate mission.

Defining Expectations of Team Members

An action-oriented team requires direction. The customer service champion should serve as the team leader, but responsibilities for leading meetings should be shared among the members. Our team created a calendar that assigned meeting leader duties and recorder duties over a 12-month period.

Ground Rules

In our organization, we follow a set of ground rules in all of our quality improvement teams. Presenting the ground rules during the first meeting sends a clear message that you have a serious task at hand and that there are expectations for each team member. Figure 3-1 presents the ground rules for teams at Watertown Area Health Services.

One responsibility of customer service team members that is not clarified in the general ground rules is that of ambassadorship. Team members will help to facilitate a culture shift by bringing the mission, goals, and plans of the customer service team forward into their individual departments. In doing so, they will be providing consistent reminders to coworkers that the customer service initiative is alive and well and reaching every corner of the organization.

Team Goals

Our group was initially established with one overriding goal in mind: to improve customer service. Once the mission was clearly stated we needed to move toward specific goals that would help us achieve that mission. This is the point where the customer service champion must serve as a facilitator and leader. A mission statement without measurable, achievable goals and a clear action plan is nothing more than a dream. The customer service champion must help that dream come to fruition by facilitating the team through specific goal development.

Goal development begins by asking the following critical questions:

- What do we (as an organization) want to achieve?
- Who do we need to reach in order to achieve our mission?
- How will we know we have arrived at our destination?
- What strengths, weaknesses, opportunities, and threats exist in relation to achieving our mission?

Brainstorming through these questions under the direction of the customer service champion as facilitator will serve as a springboard for more specific goal statements. It may take several meetings to develop specific, measurable goals. If the mission

Figure 3-1. Quality Improvement Team's Ground Rules

1. *Attendance:* Legitimate reasons to miss a meeting:
   a. Death/illness
   b. Family/department emergency
   c. External seminars/meetings as long as other arrangements have been exhausted—no substitutes
   d. Paid time off
2. *Cancellation:* If you cannot attend a meeting, notify _____ (name of leader) immediately. Alternate: _____. The meeting will be canceled when _____ (number) or more cannot attend. _____ (Leader) will notify all members of cancellation.
3. *Promptness:* Meetings will always begin and end on time. Members are expected to appear 5 minutes early to ensure a prompt start.
4. *Meeting date and time:* Team will meet _____ from _____ unless otherwise notified.
5. *Decisions/QI model:* Decisions will be by consensus. The FOCUS-PDCA model for quality improvement will be used.
6. *Interruptions:* The "100-mile" rule will be enforced. Only one conversation allowed at a time. (The 100-mile rule means that your department should treat this meeting with the same regard it would if you were attending one that is being held 100 miles away.)
7. *Role of leader:* Encourage 100 percent participation. Enforce rules. Use facilitator as needed. Leader: _____.
8. *Role of recorder:* Watch time. Take minutes. Perform meeting summary. Distribute minutes (original copy to _____ for inclusion in binder). Distribute minutes within _____ days of meeting. Rotate duties among members.
9. *Reporting mechanism:* Results will be reported to: _____.
10. *Participation:* All members must listen attentively and are expected to contribute all ideas. If issues are exhausted, enforce the "dead horse" rule.
11. *Assignments:* Assignments will be given during meetings and recorded in meeting minutes. All assignments must be completed by the agreed due date.
12. *System focus:* Members must always focus on process and system improvements. Discussion should never include attacks on personal performance.
13. *Record of activities:* _____ will retain original copies of meeting minutes in team binder.
14. *Agenda:* Team will use an agenda for all meetings. An agenda for the next meeting will be generated at the end of each meeting.
15. *Confidentiality:* All discussions in the meeting are confidential; information may be revealed only with the approval or direction of the team.

was clearly stated, the key questions listed above will guide the team into specific goals flowing naturally into the classic model—assess, plan, implement, and evaluate. Or in total quality management terms, Plan-Do-Check-Act.

In our situation, we developed the following three overriding goals under which all future actions would fall:

1. Conducting a baseline assessment of the organization in terms of customer satisfaction
2. Creating a corporatewide training program to clarify expectations and build awareness of, and support for, improved customer service at all levels
3. Establishing specific standards for customer service behavior

The steps needed for reaching each of these goals are clearly delineated in the three subsequent chapters. Chapter 4 helps the reader establish baseline information about the organization. Chapter 5 outlines the steps we at Watertown took to create standards. Chapter 6 reviews our team's steps for conducting corporatewide training sessions: creating a process, gathering support materials, and implementation.

Once these goals were achieved, we tailored the second generation of team members to meet a new set of goals and objectives. Keeping the team somewhat fluid helps to build buy-in at many levels and prevents stagnation. This issue is addressed in more detail in chapter 7.

Summary

Formation of a multidisciplinary team is the first step in building buy-in throughout the organization. Additional steps for building buy-in are covered in subsequent chapters. It is up to the customer service champion to create and lead the team, keeping it focused on the mission and helping it establish clear goals. Team members must also be clear about their responsibilities. In addition to attending meetings and helping to reach established goals, team members must view themselves as ambassadors for the cause. In order to build credibility for the initiative, team members must be the first role models for exemplary customer-focused behaviors. In addition, they have a responsibility to share team goals and progress with their respective departments. Encouraging team members to act as a liaison between the team and their departments will create a grassroots environment for change. When team members see their role as broader than the immediate tasks at hand, they become catalysts for the cultural shift.

CHAPTER FOUR

Where Are You Now?— Establishing Your Baseline

"You've got to be very careful if you don't know where you're going. Because you might not get there."
—Lawrence "Yogi" Berra

Objectives

After completing this chapter the reader will:

- Be prepared to measure baseline data

- Understand the importance of starting your service improvement plans with clear baseline data

You Are Here! But Where's Here? Imagine calling AAA and saying, "I want to go to Dallas. I need to know how long it will take to get there and the best route." The trip planner on the other end of the phone will very likely ask, "Where are you now?" If you can't give a specific location, she can't possibly give you a clear answer. She will probably instruct you to identify your coordinates and call back.

Not knowing your starting point is as detrimental as not knowing your destination. If you don't know where you are, it's difficult to get started as well as to motivate and lead others to change their behavior. This chapter will help the customer service champion gain a clearer understanding of the road map for the course that lies ahead. He or she plays the role of the navigator most of the time but occasionally that of the pilot. Like a good navigator, the customer service champion must begin by locating the organization's coordinates—in other words, the baseline data.

Gathering Baseline Data

If you haven't been measuring satisfaction, it may be difficult to motivate others to improve. After all, who says they're not doing great right now? Employees and physicians need to know how they are faring today in order to set a course for improvement over time. Just as a thorough assessment is the crucial first step in a diagnosis and treatment plan, baseline data will help you to set and reach clear, identifiable customer service goals.

Begin by taking an honest look at how your customers view the organization. The ideal assessment will include satisfaction ratings from patients, employees, and physicians.

Baseline—the Patients' Perspective

What are they saying about you? Hospitals and clinics across the country are using a multitude of tools and methods to measure patient satisfaction. The most important element in completing a solid baseline assessment is input from patients that provides credible information about their overall satisfaction and a prediction of loyalty. The second factor to consider is how the data will be compiled. Will data be accessible enough to get customized reports that will help you to zero in on specific issues? Will they be clear enough for everyone to understand?

Conducting in-house research can prove costly and cumbersome. From printing and mailing surveys to data entry and report generation, there is no doubt that gathering meaningful data is labor intensive. There are, however, advantages to conducting your own research. One of the advantages of an in-house system is that you will have access to information quickly. This can prove useful when managers want more in-depth information to help them home in on a specific problem on their units. Another advantage is that the organization can ask questions of specific concern.

Some of the disadvantages of doing your own research have already been mentioned. The labor intensity is a definite drawback. Other disadvantages include the inability to secure comparative data with other providers as well as concerns about the validity and reliability of questions. If comparative data aren't a driving concern, an in-house approach may be sufficient. But bear in mind that consumers are more sophisticated today than ever before. They seek and expect comparative information on air travel, hotel accommodations, and fast food. It is only a matter of time before comparative data on health care are widely accessed and heeded in the mainstream.

There are several reputable firms that conduct patient satisfaction research. If you are seeking an outside firm to provide a turnkey process for measuring patient satisfaction, you will want to find out how the questions were developed and tested. You may also want to know the size of the existing data repository and if comparative data can be separated into geographic region and by organization size.

Advantages of having patient satisfaction research done by an outside firm are largely dependent on the firm, its survey tool, and its methodology. Assuming that you select a credible firm with a proven track record, advantages will include credibility of comparative data, reliability, and efficiency. Cost may be a disadvantage, but many organizations find that the efficiency and reliability are worth the cost.

When choosing a firm to conduct surveys, there are some important questions to ask. Dr. Raymond Carey provides a simple reference list of both questions for the purchaser to answer and questions to pose to the survey firm.[1] He outlines the questions as follows:

- For the purchaser:
  —Why are you conducting a survey?
  —Who will use the results?
  —Will their needs be met?
- For the survey firm:
  —Is there written documentation of validity?
  —Is there written documentation of reliability?
  —Is sampling support available?
  —Has an estimate of sampling error been provided?
  —What is the expected response rate?
  —What is the report turnaround time?
  —Do the report formats meet users' needs?
  —What is the size of the database?
  —What is the quality of the database?
  —Is there flexibility in adding questions?

Your selection of a firm should take these issues as well as cost into consideration.

Baseline—the Employees' Perspective

Employee satisfaction surveys are another important element of establishing your baseline. Employees are the internal customers whose opinions are shaped by (but also help to shape) the corporate culture. By assessing employee satisfaction, you will be identifying the internal strengths, weaknesses, and opinions that will either help or hinder goals for service excellence.

Similar to patient satisfaction, there are advantages and disadvantages to conducting your own surveys. Advantages include survey process and results that are ongoing and the ability to modify questions to address current issues. However, employees are often more than a little paranoid that their responses will get back to the manager or administration. Hiring an outside firm may help to quell these fears. Again, there are many reputable firms that conduct employee satisfaction surveys. At Watertown Area Health Services, we found it advantageous to work with a company that could add questions that would help us to home in on specific areas of concern. In doing so, we had the advantage of comparative data but with a few additional questions that were customized for our needs. We intentionally added questions about the effectiveness of 12 information sources used within our organization. By adding these questions, we were able to determine the best method for communicating the results of the survey.

When introducing the idea of employee satisfaction surveys in our organization we heard some grumbling. There seemed to be a prevailing attitude that "we've done that, and nothing ever comes of it. Why tell administration what's wrong if nothing ever changes?" There was also distrust that candid remarks would be used against them.

In order to achieve the level of participation needed at Watertown, administration had to set the stage with a promise that we would publish the results and keep employees informed about decisions made and actions taken as a result of the survey. Even though there was some initial skepticism, over time we have built up confidence in the fact that the information was openly shared and used to design change. We also shifted to using an in-house tool distributed every 90 days with payroll. Although we process the surveys internally, we have an outside vendor that provides benchmarks for industry comparisons.

Baseline—the Medical Staff's Perspective

The medical staff is another crucially important customer group. Its members' opinions of the organization's operations, facilities, administration, and staff can have a direct influence on patient satisfaction as well as on medical staff longevity with your hospital. Listening to this group can help give you a picture of the problems as well as strengths inherent in your organization. Again, you will need to choose between an outside firm and an internal format for your assessment, and there are advantages and disadvantages to both. The medical staff is a smaller sample than employees and patients and therefore may be more manageable for in-house staff. The challenge in using an internal method is the survey design and statistical analysis. Unless you have a professional who is proficient in these functions, the results may be questionable. Physicians by nature are empirical thinkers schooled in the scientific process. Of all the groups with whom you work, they are the most likely to question your method and the data's validity, reliability, and statistical significance. At Watertown, we were fortunate to have the in-house expertise to design a survey that was not only useful but defensible. As with the employees, we stressed our commitment to communicating results and taking action to improve areas of concern.

Measuring our physicians' satisfaction helped us set specific and measurable goals for improvement. Building loyalty among members of the medical staff as well as credibility for the rest of our customer service efforts meant that we had to demonstrate our commitment to acting on the information gathered. The data proved to be a springboard from which we made several important changes. It was also useful to the employees to see how physician satisfaction with one department or service could be closely correlated with their overall satisfaction with, and loyalty to, the organization.

Seeing the Big Picture

Once completed, the three assessments—patients', employees', and medical staff's—will help to paint a picture of your organization's strengths, weaknesses, opportunities, and threats. Analyze the information to identify strengths and weaknesses. Once the strengths are identified, you will be able to plan strategies to capitalize on them. Weaknesses should be identified and acted on quickly. But change cannot occur if this information is kept secret. Share the information among the internal groups in the spirit of healthy change. The goal is not to point fingers but to craft solutions. We made a conscious effort to share summaries of the results of our baseline assessment with each separate group but also between groups as well. For instance, all employees were exposed, not only to the results of the employee survey, but also to the patient satisfaction data and physician opinion survey. Physicians saw the patient and employee satisfaction data as well as the results of their medical staff survey. In order to ensure confidentiality of the survey participants, we didn't share verbatim comments. Confidentiality was promised and strictly adhered to throughout the process.

Department managers were able to use the information from all three surveys to help craft their respective departments' customer service action plans (see chapter 8).

Summary

Collecting and analyzing baseline data are as crucial to the future of your customer service efforts as a thorough examination is to a physician's diagnosis and treatment plan. But data are only as good as the strategies that arise from them. In the following chapters, you will begin to see how you can consistently use data to reinforce the positive as well as to isolate and act on the negative. A solid baseline of information at this stage will help to build buy-in during the training sessions. When staff can see statistical evidence of customers' perceptions, they are much more likely to accept the importance of customer service throughout the organization.

Reference

1. Raymond G. Carey, "How to Choose a Patient Survey System," *Journal on Quality Improvement* 25, no. 1 (January 1999): 22.

CHAPTER FIVE

Creating Meaningful Standards to Live By

"You can't 'policy' people's hearts."
—Quint Studer, CEO,
Baptist Hospital, Pensacola, FL

Objectives

After completing this chapter the reader will:

- Have the tools to identify stellar performers within the organization and enlist their support in drafting standards

- Be able to clearly state behaviors associated with good customer service

- Be able to create custom-made standards unique to your organization

I open this chapter with the quote from Quint Studer for good reason. The logic inherent in the words epitomizes the rationale for setting standards. Consistent, clearly communicated standards will help foster a more desirable culture. Trying to create policies or mandates won't change people's hearts, but a grassroots approach to standards development may help to foster a more desirable culture. This chapter guides the reader through a process designed to develop meaningful standards for the organization. By following the suggested process, the customer service champion will be building buy-in for the customer service initiative while gaining valuable insights into the core values of stellar performers within the organization.

Why Create Standards for Customer Service Performance?

Defining standards creates a baseline for everyone in the organization. By clarifying expectations, you are helping to make service-oriented behavior a fundamental requirement for employment. Placing expectations in writing provides a consistent reminder for each employee and measurable criteria by which managers can evaluate individual performance. And once the standards have been communicated, distributed, and posted, none of the employees can say they didn't know what was expected. Ideally, the customer service standards will be included as a section of each employee's annual review or evaluation.

Who Should Define the Standards?

That is a question that will be unique to each organization involved in the customer service improvement process. In our situation at Watertown, we sought input from individuals recognized for exemplary performance. We gathered them together, picked their brains about service excellence, and coached them through the process of identifying specific behaviors associated with abstract qualities. Beginning with focus groups, we worked with more than 20 individuals to define our standards. We found the process to be very effective and by involving star performers we were able to create instant credibility for the standards.

Look for Role Models

Everyone has role models—people whom they admire for their personality, outlook on life, or people skills. I feel confident that if you ask around your organization, you will find service heroes in nearly every nook and corner who are already serving as role models for others. You need only ask who they are, and you'll have no problem finding them. Our team at Watertown decided that rather than having us define service standards for the staff to follow, we should consult the real experts on customer service in our organization—the heroes in the trenches who were admired by others for their skills, compassion, and common sense.

By turning to our internal role models as resources for customer service standards, we accomplished the following three objectives:

1. We expanded the circle of influence of the customer service team.
2. We tapped into the existing culture of the organization.
3. We helped to boost buy-in by having standards designed by the people who had already been identified as stellar performers by their peers, managers, and patients.

In their book *The Real Heroes of Business,* Bill Fromm and Len Schlesinger state:

> If you want to know how to give great customer service, find people who do it and watch them work. If you want to keep

great customer service performers in your company, find people who are great service performers, and ask them what's important to them, how they like to be managed, and what makes them happy in their work.[1]

Our approach to identifying customer service heroes in our organization was fairly simple. We tapped into three logical sources for names: patient satisfaction surveys, managers' referrals, and winners of the employee-of-the-month program (a program, incidentally, no longer in existence).

Patient satisfaction surveys are a logical source for identifying stellar performers. When patients are extremely impressed with an individual during their stay, they will often single that individual out in comments on their satisfaction survey. Acts of extraordinary kindness, efficiency, or skill do not go unnoticed at our organization. Our CEO makes a point of sending personal letters to employees named by patients in their survey comments. He not only takes the time to write thank-you letters, but also sends them to their homes so that their families will know how much they are appreciated. Copies are also sent to the employees' managers and one is added to their personnel files so the managers can publicly praise the employees.

When selecting members for our focus group, the CEO's correspondence file became a wellspring of information on exceptional performers. Going back over a one-year period, we were able to identify several individuals who had been commended anywhere from one to twelve times by patients.

We had to be cautious, however, that we didn't focus only on individuals identified in patient satisfaction surveys, because by doing so we would risk targeting only those involved in direct patient care. Keeping in mind that customer service heroes were as important in materials management, dietary services, the business office, and housekeeping as they are at the bedside, we found two additional sources for names.

At that time, our hospital had an employee-of-the-month program. Each month, an award was bestowed on an individual identified by coworkers as a stellar example of customer service. Although I had some personal misgivings about the concept of employee-of-the-month in general, it did provide a source for names that were clearly role models for other employees. (I later identified my resistance to the program to the fact that it had never been linked to specific standards or values. This is addressed in more detail in chapter 7.)

The third source we turned to was the management staff. Having recently completed annual performance evaluations, managers had renewed insight into customer service heroes in their respective departments.

Make It Their Idea

Each of us has a need to feel that our suggestions and ideas are valued. And when we feel valued, we are much more likely to work harder for the person or organization that openly appreciates our value. In his book *The Corporate Coach,* James Miller states, "People work hardest to achieve ideas that they believe in. And not surprisingly, people have the strongest belief in their own ideas."[2]

Operating with this view in mind, we began talking with the outstanding performers of our organization about their beliefs, values, and how they approach their jobs every day. Groups of 10 to 12 employees were organized into focus groups with specific objectives. I use the term *focus group* for these discussions while realizing that the methodology may not fit with the strict scientific approach to research.

The following steps were taken to craft the focus groups to give the most meaningful results.

Focus Group Objectives and Discussion Guide

A well-run focus group begins with defining objectives. Our overall objective for the initial focus group was to get the group members to identify the customer service qualities that have made them stand out in our hospital. The second objective was to get them talking about the culture of the organization and whether they felt a customer service initiative would be effective and why or why not.

Preparation for the group requires setting clear objectives that will drive the discussion. Once the objectives are clarified, the moderator can design questions that will meet the objectives. The questions serve merely as a guide. Every focus group is as different as its participants are. The goal is to get participants talking about the identified issues and delving into their responses for deeper meaning.

Once the moderator's questions were drafted, the outline was presented to our customer service team for feedback. Members of the team had the opportunity to review key questions and make suggestions for additions or changes. This step helps to keep the process in sync with the customer service team's mission and goals. It also helps the team members feel more involved in the process.

The following is a sample of the questions covered in our first focus group, along with some of the responses.

- When you think of a company known for its customer service, which one comes to mind? What makes you say that?
- How do you think these companies developed their reputations?
- How do you define customers? *Anyone who has expectations of us or needs that are met by us.*
- Who are our customers? *Patients, families, visitors, physicians, coworkers, payers, clergy, and vendors.*
- Can we divide the customer list into internal and external? *Coworkers are internal customers. The rest are external.*
- What do you think each of these groups of customers expects from us? *Internal customers expect respect, conflict resolution,*

responsibility, integrity, a positive attitude, and teamwork. External customers expect personalized care, prompt attention, professionalism, respect, privacy, and clear information.

- If you were in charge of customer service, how would you let employees know what you expect from them in terms of customer service? *Training and standards for performance.*
- How would you handle employees who do not follow your prescribed customer service behaviors? *Additional training, discipline, and termination.*

The discussion up to this point typically takes over an hour. Here the moderator summarized the discussion by reviewing the key points we had listed on flip chart sheets. In our focus groups at Watertown, I reviewed the information and offered to summarize the notes from the discussion and distribute them to participants. The participants were invited back to continue the discussion after one week. Their assignment was to review the summary and to begin thinking of specific behaviors that demonstrate how to meet customer expectations. The second discussion was directed at identifying specific behaviors that we wanted to demonstrate.

Conducting Focus Groups

The success of a focus group can be greatly enhanced by giving some forethought to the room setup and materials. The following section offers pointers for setting up group discussions that will make participants feel welcome and keep them involved.

Scheduling the Groups

In hospital settings where people work around the clock, it is important to schedule options that will allow participation from all three shifts. Early morning and midafternoon seemed to be the most convenient times for our participants. You will need the following items:

- *Flip chart* to record key concepts
- *Tape* to tape up pages from the flip chart
- *Markers* for writing on the flip chart
- *Name plates* to identify participants to one another

Select a desirable setting. Choose a quiet room with a large table where, when seated, all participants can see one another and the moderator, who will be standing with the flip chart. Serve light refreshments (perhaps coffee and muffins in the morning, cookies and soda in the afternoon).

Extending a Welcome

The customer service champion can serve as the focus group moderator and should set the stage for the focus group by being there when participants first arrive. Greeting the participants and inviting them to help themselves to food and beverages help to set a relaxed, casual atmosphere. As participants arrive, hand them a name plate (an index card folded in half lengthwise works well) and ask them to place it in front of them on the table.

Setting the Ground Rules

Stating the ground rules in the beginning is an important first step. When working with groups of employees, I find it necessary to stress that they all participate candidly and that one of the expectations is that the discussions remain confidential. I let them know that I will be sharing a summary of the discussion with the administrative team as well as with the customer service team, but the summary will capture only the essence of the discussion and not the details of what was said by whom. The following is a list of some general ground rules I present at the beginning of the discussions.

- Names of participants are confidential. I ask that each of you respect one another's right to speak out and share ideas without fear that your words will be shared outside this room.
- Notes are being taken by my assistant because I have a lousy memory, and rather than trying to write a million miles an hour, I can just look at notes.
- A summary will be compiled of what was said, but not by whom. The summary will be shared with the customer service team.
- One person should speak at a time. You have been provided with a notepad in which to jot down ideas if someone else is talking.
- Avoid side conversations—I don't want to miss any of the good stuff.
- All opinions are of value here even if they differ from others. This meeting is about an exchange of ideas, not a consensus.
- There are no right or wrong answers here.
- Session length is $1\frac{1}{2}$ hours.
- I have two expectations for each of you: that you participate and that you speak candidly.

Summarizing the Results

After all the sessions are completed, summarize the information into a succinct report with recommendations. At Watertown, our recommendation was to continue working with the same group of stellar performers in drafting the standards and testing the training format.

After the initial focus groups were completed, the participants were asked to join the task force for two to three meetings. Task force participants knew at the start of the second meeting that the goal of our task force was to end up with a deliverable document that would serve as a set of standards for customer service performance for every person in the organization. That goal was set as a result of input at the first meeting when participants expressed a desire to clarify standards for employees. At the conclusion of our discussions we would have a set of standards that would be presented to all employees within the organization.

Later, when the standards were presented to the managers and staff during the corporatewide training sessions, the names of the focus group participants were listed (with their permission). We felt it was important to publicly recognize these individuals as the experts behind the document. In doing this, we would be spotlighting the people that we wanted others to imitate. We would be making the statement that the standards were not created by administrators, whom many thought were too removed from the realities of the departments, but by their peers who work with them in the trenches every day.

Moving from Discussion to Specific Behaviors

The second and third meetings with the task force were geared toward identifying specific desirable behaviors. This process required moving from discussing customer service in generalities to discussing specific behaviors. Pinpointing behaviors requires a skilled moderator. One of the most crucial skills is that of probing. During discussions when participants identify a quality, the moderator will need to help the group to identify the specific behaviors elicited that depict that quality. For example, group members easily identified courtesy as one of their common traits. The challenge for them was in identifying behaviors that our customers associate with courtesy. The typical discussions went something like this:

> *Moderator (M):* Let's talk about what qualities you all have that have made you stand out as stellar performers in this organization. Give me some examples of your unique qualities. (List all the responses offered, then return to the list to begin delving in more depth.)

Participant (P): Courtesy. I try to always be courteous.

M: When you say courteous, what does that mean?

P: Well, it means that I'm polite and respectful.

M: What does that look like? If I were trying to break down the word *courteous* into specific actions, what would I actually see you do?

P: Well, I always greet people by name. I say "please" and "thank you."

At the conclusion of this discussion, the customer service champion will have the first draft of what will later become the working document. Not everyone is a writer, so trying to finalize a document as a group is too laborious. I recommend that the customer service champion summarize the discussion into a list of qualities and associated behaviors for the group's review at the next meeting. The process may need to be repeated a few times before the group feels that their suggestions are accurately presented.

Figure 5-1 is the final draft of the standards developed by our stellar performers. Each employee received a copy of the standards during the training sessions. They were later posted in every department within the hospital and at each affiliated service or satellite. Figure 5-2 presents the thank-you letter sent to each focus group participant.

Summary

Creating standards is an essential step in clarifying corporate-wide expectations for behavior. By involving stellar performers from all levels and disciplines within the organization, the customer service champion will be fostering the grassroots focus. At the conclusion of this step, the customer service team will have one of the core elements needed in the training sessions.

Figure 5-1. Customer Service Standards and Pledge

Internal Customers: Our pledge to each other (fellow employees and hospital personnel)

"Respect me and my job."

Our need: Respect.

Our response: I understand the need to be respected, and I will:

- Acknowledge you
- Be sensitive to your point of view
- Thank you for a job well done
- Value your time and priorities
- Discuss my concerns with you in private
- Value your job and its contribution to the organization
- Treat you as I would like to be treated
- Speak to you in a pleasant tone in person or on the phone

"We are all professionals."

Our need: Professionalism

Our response: I understand the need to represent Watertown Memorial Hospital in a professional manner, and I will:

- Take responsibility for my actions
- Protect confidential information about patients or fellow employees
- Look professional in dress, grooming, and manner
- Coach others when necessary
- Follow through on my promise to you

"Work/communicate with me."

Our need: Teamwork.

Our response: I understand the need for teamwork, and I will:

- Pitch in and offer to help you whenever possible
- Ask for your input before making a decision that may affect you
- Talk to you directly instead of talking to others secretly if I have a concern
- Listen to you, offer positive advice, and not interrupt until you are finished
- Recognize that everyone has a valid opinion
- Seek out information and share what I have learned

"Smile—it's contagious!"

Our need: Positive attitude

Our response: I understand the need for a positive work environment, and I will:

- Be sensitive to the effects my actions have on others
- Replace criticism with positive ideas
- Try to see things through the other person's eyes
- Attempt to leave my personal problems at home
- Coach my coworkers in portraying a positive attitude
- Project a caring and concerned attitude

Figure 5-2. Customer Service Participant Thank-You Letter

Dear _____

A few weeks ago you participated in some discussions to help us develop a customer service program at WMH. Your input is greatly appreciated and I wanted to let you know how your ideas are being put to good use.

- The managers received a summary of your ideas and suggestions at the March management information meeting.
- The customer service team is using your ideas to develop a training program with three audiences in mind: new employees, managers, and existing employees.
- The customer service team is planning to begin the new program in June.

We'd appreciate your feedback on the new training program before we offer it to all employees. We will be contacting you in the future with a date and location for the preview.

Thank you again for your time and input. It's amazing what we can accomplish when we all put our heads together.

Sincerely,

Kris Baird

References

1. Bill Fromm and Len Schlesinger, *The Real Heroes of Business: And Not a CEO among Them* (New York: Currency Doubleday, 1993), p. xviii.

2. James Miller, *The Corporate Coach* (New York: St. Martin's Press, 1993), p. 107.

CHAPTER SIX

The Training Sessions—
Getting Everyone
on the Same Page

Objectives

After completing this chapter the reader will:

- Be prepared to assist the CEO in setting the stage for the training sessions

- Be prepared to conduct corporatewide training sessions tailored to specific audiences

- Recognize the importance of using several different teaching methods during the training sessions

- Have a sample agenda and materials for training sessions targeting managers, newly hired employees, and long-term employees

In 1997 Watertown Area Health Services introduced a branding campaign that would unify our hospital with its rural satellite clinics, community-based residential facilities, and home health agency. As in many other organizations, there was a media campaign surrounding the introduction of the new corporate identity. While this is essential for enhancing recognition, we also wanted to instill a sense of pride among our employees that the logo represented more than the corporate entity. We wanted every person seeing that logo to associate it with excellent customer service. In order to accomplish that goal, we had to make certain that every employee understood the customer service team's and administration's expectations for customer service. Corporatewide training sessions held over a four-week period allowed us to introduce the customer service standards and clarify expectations, first for managers, then for the entire staff.

This chapter offers guidelines for setting up training objectives for each individual group within your organization. The training example presented here uses several different teaching methods in order to hold the participants' interest and attention. Designed to appeal to individuals of all educational levels, the training agenda is objective driven. By following this format, you will be laying the groundwork for future efforts.

Seek First to Understand, Then to Be Understood

Operating under this credo, customer service training becomes a simple matter of stepping into someone else's shoes. Our customer service team identified that there were very specific groups within our organization that had unique needs and responsibilities, which had to be understood in order for the team to set meaningful objectives for the training sessions as well as job descriptions and evaluation criteria pertinent to customer service. The administration, middle managers, long-term employees, and new hires were the four groups we identified as having unique needs relative to our goal of fostering a culture of customer service excellence. Other hospitals, clinics, or systems may have fewer, some more. Table 6-1, a Customer Service Planning Guide, offers an overview of the four unique groups with their responsibilities to the organization and their training needs and objectives.

The medical staff is a group unto itself. From the very first customer service training session and for months to come, the staff at Watertown persisted in asking, "What about the physicians? Aren't they just as important in this process as we are?" The answer to that question is an unequivocal yes. The caveat, however, is that they function somewhat independently of the employees and require not only their own set of rules, but a unique action plan. For this reason, I have addressed the medical staff separately in chapter 8.

The following pages will help to distinguish key learning needs and differences between groups within your organization. Once specific groups have been identified, you can begin to list their unique learning needs and specific tactics for addressing those needs. When trying to differentiate specific groups, consider the following questions:

- What is the group's main role within the organization (leader, supervisor, line staff)?
- Does this group of individuals have direct contact with the public and/or patients?
- Are they responsible for hiring, supervising, training, or evaluating others?
- What is their circle of influence? How do coworkers perceive them (leader, role model, or authority)?
- How long have they been with the organization (new hires versus established employees)?
- Who are their key customers (patients, payers, physicians, coworkers)?

Answering these questions helps define different groups within the organization. This is crucial because as you proceed with an action plan, you must distinguish unique needs and challenges in order to craft your message and objectives.

Table 6-1. Customer Service Planning Guide

Group	Responsibilities	Needs	Training Objective
Administration	• Lead the organization • Communicate missión and vision • Clarify expectations • Build a strong layer of middle managers • Hold managers accountable • Serve as role models	• Craft a message that clarifies expectations of managers and staff • Tie customer service to performance evaluations	• Demonstrate a unified position on the importance of customer service (CS) as a corporate objective • Reinforce managers' accountability for enforcing CS at all levels • Hold managers accountable for their departmental goals and related satisfaction scores • Incorporate CS standards into managers' job descriptions and annual review
Managers	• Hire, train, and support staff • Monitor, mentor, and evaluate staff performance • Serve as role models • Manage depart-ments for quality performance and fiscal responsibility	• Understand the managers' role in training and mentoring staff in customer service performance	• Understand the WMH CS philosophy and the management role in fostering a corporate culture of CS • Preview corporate training program including standards • Demonstrate personal accountability for CS by setting measurable departmental goals and clear standards for per-formance associated with each job description • Recognize the importance of ongoing emphasis on CS in daily operations • Understand how to lead the department in setting goals and creating a customer service action plan • Gain skills that enable them to foster a sound customer service philosophy through role-modeling, education, coaching, and feedback

Table 6-1. (Continued)

Group	Responsibilities	Needs	Training Objective
Long-term employees	• Perform duties according to defined expectations • Demonstrate behaviors consistent with standards	• Understand how customer service fits with corporate values, vision, and goals	• Understand CS standards and corporate-wide expectations for associated behaviors • Understand personal accountability for performing according to established CS standards • Understand consequences for noncompliance with the established standards
New hires	• Learn what is expected in their new job	• Understand how customer service fits with corporate values, vision, and goals • Be exposed to customer service as a priority in the corporate culture	• Understand CS standards and corporate-wide expectations • Understand personal accountability for performing according to established CS standards

One Size Doesn't Fit All—Understanding Unique Training Needs

Table 6-2 illustrates the differences in training needs between managers and staff. While both groups need to understand the importance of customer service standards, managers have the additional role of monitoring, measuring, and reinforcing behaviors. Their accountability for staff performance and customer satisfaction creates a unique set of training needs. For this reason, I recommend a separate training session for managers and supervisors that stresses the need for corporatewide performance standards and the manager's responsibility for holding staff to those standards. Management training sessions should be held about one week before launching the staff training sessions. This offers managers a sneak preview of the

Table 6-2. Goals, Training Tactics, and Objectives

Segment	Program Goals	Tactics	Objectives
New employees	All new employees will understand and practice a sound customer service (CS) philosophy To present clear expectations for customer service to new employees during the orientation process	• Administrator presents "who are our customers" to new orientees • Show videotapes on customer service • Distribute standards pledge cards	• Understand the 16 standards of excellence in customer service • Receive and review the standards pledge cards • Understand how to interact with all customer groups according to standards • Understand the WMH process for conflict resolution
Management	The management team will gain a clear understanding of the customer service philosophy and training program by —— The management team will foster a sound customer service philosophy through role-modeling, education, coaching, and feedback	• Attend a management training session to introduce corporate training program • View videos and complete workbooks associated with training program • Meet with department staff to define customers and related service issues • Set clear departmental CS goals with staff • Report departments' CS goals to management team	• Understand the WMH CS philosophy and the management role in fostering a corporate culture of CS • Demonstrate personal accountability for CS by setting measurable departmental goals and clear standards for performance associated with each job description • Recognize the importance of ongoing emphasis on CS in daily operations

Table 6-2. (Continued)

Segment	Program Goals	Tactics	Objectives
Existing employees	All WMH employees will understand and practice a sound customer service philosophy All WMH employees will attend a CS training session and receive a copy of CS standards by	• Will attend mandatory training sessions	• Understand CS standards and corporatewide expectations • Understand personal accountability for performing according to established CS standards • Understand consequences for non-compliance with the established standards
Customer service team	To create and foster a sound customer service philosophy throughout WMH and its affiliated services	• Define standards for customer service excellence • Define segments, learning needs, and tactics unique to each segment • Prepare curriculum and time line for implementation, including launch and follow-up	

training materials being shared with staff and helps them to see the importance of promoting staff attendance.

Management Training

The overriding goal for the management training session is to emphasize the need for consistent, visible leadership from the managers on a daily basis that will reinforce customer service behaviors among their subordinates. In addition to offering exemplary customer service themselves, managers must reinforce positive staff behavior and work to modify negative behavior. But unless managers hear this message from the CEO, along with plans for evaluating their performance related to customer service, they may not take it seriously. Managers also need to hear that administration will support them in their role and will offer additional training and coaching where needed. It is unfair for an administrative team to spell out expectations and then not provide the tools to help the managers succeed.

Managers in particular need to address the issue of customer service in terms of their role as leaders. Marsha Borling stresses that one of the core reasons that provider organizations do not achieve excellence is that "intolerable service is tolerated."[1]

When asked how to enlighten managers on this issue, Borling stated:

> The change has to start at the top. The leadership must clarify expectations of its managers, then provide them with the tools and support needed to build a customer-sensitive work environment. Then comes the tough part: holding them accountable. If you tell managers that meeting and exceeding customer needs is an expectation, then you have to let them know how you will be measuring and fostering their growth as managers.
>
> One core expectation for management is that they measure and monitor staff performance related to customer service excellence. Help managers to recognize that monitoring employees' approach to customer service is just as important as monitoring and controlling drug errors or safety breaches.

When managers are inconsistent or unfair in their enforcement of customer service expectations, they quickly erode a department's morale.[2]

Tie the Message to Existing Policy

The management training session offers a great opportunity to review disciplinary action policy and procedure as well as techniques for confronting difficult employees. Avoiding confrontation is a common reason that many managers don't deal with problem behavior. They may need reassurance that the disciplinary policies can be a great help in redirecting behavior. In our organization a series of verbal and written warnings are issued prior to suspension or dismissal. Reviewing the procedure and role-playing through an actual case example can be helpful for managers who have never used the formal disciplinary protocol. We incorporated such a section in our management training module and found it to be quite effective.

Our CEO kicked off the program with a very strong, encouraging statement, recreated in figure 6-1, about his expectations for the managers. He linked his remarks to the hospital's mission and vision. Figure 6-2 provides an overview of our management training session.

It is important for senior leadership to take a public stand regarding expectations for the management and staff. For that reason, an administrative team needs to be a very visible part of the training sessions. Prior to the actual training sessions, the customer service champion should meet with the CEO and senior leadership team to discuss their role in the training sessions. Our team felt that opening the training sessions with a statement by the administrator would give credibility to the rest of the program. We defined the administrative team's role as follows:

- To demonstrate a unified position on the importance of customer service as a corporate objective

Figure 6-1. Manager Training—CEO's Opening Statements

Corporatewide Expectations and Personal Accountability

If we stay focused on one key goal, the importance of customer service is crystal clear. We want WMH to be a place where patients want to be treated, physicians want to practice, and employees want to work. Excellence in customer service is the surest, straightest path toward that goal. The board and administrative team recognize the importance of this customer service initiative and are in full support of the team's efforts. Today's session will clarify our expectations of you and offer tools to ensure that you have what you need to make it happen.

What we expect of managers and coordinators:

- To be leaders and role models. First to understand what is expected, then to teach, coach, and reinforce customer-focused behaviors from your employees.
- To lead your departments in developing a list of customers, their needs, and your action plan for enhancing your service to them.
- To be personally accountable for customer service in your area and to hold each employee accountable for performing according to the established standards.
- To confront problem behaviors promptly, professionally, and according to the processes recognized by WMH policy.

Today you will be introduced to the new customer service standards along with other tools developed to enhance customer service throughout WMH and its affiliated services. This is the groundwork for future efforts but is in no way the final product. This is a process. A living initiative that isn't as short-lived as a program or as finite as a single year's goal. As long as we are in health care, customer service must remain at the core of every encounter.

How CS pertains to your review (departmental goals):

As you know, the new performance evaluation has a strong CS component. Service quality and teamwork are two of four main categories in the new performance review process. Therefore, each of us is expected to create and implement an action plan aimed at improving customer service in our respective areas of influence.

Administrative support:

I speak on behalf of all the administrative team when I say that we are committed to raising the level of customer service at WMH. None of us has all the answers, but we're here to support you in clarifying and reaching your departmental goals.

Your main role is in translating the customer service standards into performance expectations in your areas. We will provide you with the tools and the support, but you must live the effort every day in order to make WMH a place patients want to be treated, physicians want to practice, and employees want to work.

Figure 6-2. Manager Training Agenda

I. **Introduction (presented by the CEO)**

Core values and how they pertain to customer service
Standards for performance
Expectations for managers

1. To be leaders and role models. Understand what is expected, then teach, coach, and reinforce customer-focused behaviors from your staff.
2. To lead your departments in developing a list of customers, their needs, and an action plan to address those needs.
3. To be personally accountable for customer service in your area and to hold each employee accountable for performing according to established standards.
4. To confront problem behaviors promptly, professionally, and according to the processes outlined in WMH policy.

II. **Why Customer Service?**

Overview [from chapter 1]
Marketing ladder [figure 1-1]. Positive word of mouth is based on experience
The cost of a bad experience
What our baseline data indicate
Patient satisfaction scores
Employee satisfaction scores
Physician satisfaction scores
Excerpts from focus groups—parents of pediatric patients share positive and negative experiences at WMH

III. **Customer Service Standards**

The new standards
How standards were created (input from our own stellar performers)
Using standards to guide staff
Bringing the standards back to your staff

IV. **Tools to Support Managers**

Addressing problem behaviors (presented by human resources director)
Human resources
What support is available?
Review disciplinary action policy and procedure
Documentation
Rewards, recognition, and merit pay
Confronting difficult employees (presented by EAP director)
Role-play confrontation skills
Using the EAP as a resource
Mediation services available through EAP
Personality profile (activity)
Videos that will be shown to staff: *Customer Service in Healthcare, Respect*

V. **Action Plans**

Template for departmental action plans
Using quarterly data to set goals and monitor trends

- To reinforce managers' accountability for enforcing customer service at all levels
- To follow up with managers on their departmental goals
- To incorporate customer service standards into managers' job descriptions and annual review

Keep It Interesting

Research shows that adult learners will retain more information if a variety of teaching methods are used. Our training sessions incorporated lecture, discussion, role-play, video, and experiential activities. A variety of speakers conducted the presentation, many of whom were the managers' peers, but all were employees of the organization. Changing speakers helped to maintain interest and demonstrated that the program incorporated input from a wide variety of individuals within the organization. We specifically created a homegrown program for managers and staff because we didn't want our coworkers to think the training program was a "flavor-of-the-month" fad that would disappear as rapidly as a guest speaker or consultant.

Presenting a balance of empirical data and a clear statement of values sets the stage for the management training session. There is something impersonal about seeing statistics presented. Managers and staff often have a tendency to "explain away" the reasons for poor satisfaction scores. It's not unusual to have to battle skepticism from staff and managers about these data. Convincing them to take the satisfaction data seriously can be difficult, but not impossible, and using reliable, valid measurement tools is essential. Presenting the data in a clear and meaningful fashion is also imperative. However, when I realized that we continued to battle skepticism at Watertown after an entire year of presenting satisfaction data, I had to find a new method for getting the message across. I wanted managers to see that this stuff was real and damaging to the organization. Some managers were still "explaining away" the data, so I tried to make the data more real. During the management training session I played excerpts from tapes recorded during focus groups held with former patients and community members. Without breaching confidentiality, I was able to let the managers hear the voices of their customers. When managers heard voices of parents of pediatric patients in a candid discussion about their experiences at our hospital, the data suddenly had a human element. Their stories made a strong and lasting impression on the managers about staff, services, and processes within their own departments. I highly recommend using such material if it is available. If tapes are not available, recent survey comments can also be quite telling. Be certain to share both the positive and negative comments.

Role-playing skits helped to present serious material in a light and humorous manner. Customer service team members played a variety of manager responses to challenging staff members. In one skit the manager chose to ignore a coworker's complaint about another employee's rude behavior saying, "That's just her. She's always a little testy." In another example the manager became defensive saying, "So what do you want me to do about it? I've got an entire floor to run here. I don't have time for your petty fights." In the final example, the manager listened carefully and coached the concerned employee through scenarios that would help her confront her rude coworker and open options for further discussion. While presented in a humorous manner, many of the examples helped managers to see a little of themselves.

The management training session concluded with a preview of the training program that would be offered to all staff and a directive to reconvene within one month after the last training session to present all the departments' action plans. Figure 6-3 presents an agenda for the follow-up management education meeting. A format for the departmental customer service action plan (figure 6-4) was also provided to each department. In order to prepare the plan, each manager was directed to facilitate meetings in which staff would identify

Figure 6-3. Management Education Meeting Agenda

Management Education Meeting

Goal: The goal of this meeting is to provide managers with an opportunity to share ideas related to defined customer service initiatives and to build on the momentum started with the employee training sessions.

Agenda

Why customer service?	Kris Baird
What our data show	
Targets to improve loyalty	
What is expected of managers	John Kosanovich
Review from June meeting	
Department plans	Laverne Schauer
Small-group discussions of goals, plans	
Identify similarities	
Identify ways in which we can help	
one another to achieve identified goals	
Groups share information	Laverne Schauer
Attendance at mandatory in-service	Jan Triplett
Ideas for handling attendance issues	
Next steps	Jan Triplett
Suggestions from managers	

their customers and customers' core concerns and needs and set goals to meet the defined needs. Each manager was encouraged to appoint a lead person within the department to help coordinate the department meetings and prepare the final action plan. (Action plans are discussed in more detail in chapter 7.)

Rethink the New-Employee Orientation

New employees are perhaps the easiest group to influence because they have no previous experience with the corporate culture. Of course, that is assuming that you have screened applicants carefully and hired only those who demonstrate

Figure 6-4. Departmental Customer Service Action Plan

Department _____

Date of staff meeting _____ Names of individuals attending _____

Team leader _____ (department may choose to identify a customer service champion to oversee departmental efforts)

Show *Your Co-workers as Customers* video

Identify your key customers and their needs.

Customer group	Their primary needs	What we are currently doing to meet these needs	How we can improve the way we meet customer needs	How will we know if our efforts are working? We will measure our results by:

good people skills to begin with. Common characteristics of newly hired employees include the following:

- A desire to learn about the organization
- A desire to have boundaries, ground rules, and expectations clarified as a starting point
- A need to fit in and be part of the team

Our new employees and volunteers attend a day-long orientation program to learn important information ranging from safety drills to campus tours. Because customer service is so highly regarded in our organization, it is the second message new employees hear just after the vision and mission. By following the CEO's welcoming remarks and statement of mission and vision, the new employees gain a clear understanding of where customer service fits into their new roles.

Training objectives for new employees are fairly straightforward. They include the following:

- Define the mission and vision of the organization.
- State the importance of customer satisfaction in the organization.
- Define how we measure customer satisfaction.
- Link new employees' roles in the organization with customer service and overall patient satisfaction.
- Define customer service standards.
- Define how customer service standards relate to employees' performance reviews.

By stating this information clearly on an employee's first day of work, the employer has the opportunity to clarify expectations for behavior consistent with the mission and vision of the organization. The CEO or customer service champion can deliver the message as part of every new-employee orientation. In addition to the message on mission and vision in his orientation remarks, our CEO challenges new employees to use their fresh set of senses to help us improve the working environment. He states, "You come to this organization with a fresh set of senses. You may hear, see, smell, or feel things that those of us who have been here awhile have become oblivious to. Use your newness to help us identify things about our environment that could be better. When you see, hear, smell, or feel things that could be improved, tell us. Talk to your manager or call me directly. We encourage your feedback and observations."

An outline of the customer service section of the new-employee orientation is included in figure 6-5.

After one month, we bring new employees back for a luncheon session where we review the standards and assess their perceptions of the corporate culture. Led by the customer service champion, these meetings are designed to reinforce our commitment to customer service throughout the organization and to gain insights from the new employees. Following up with the CEO's challenge to use their newness to help the organization, we talk about areas they are puzzled by and suggestions they have for improvement. We have found that new employees exposed to the standards early in their employment take them very seriously. But regardless of the convincing presentation on orientation day, credibility will quickly erode if the new employee hears this information only to witness contradictory behavior from managers and other employees. To be successful, the customer service initiative must permeate all levels consistently. For this reason, we implemented a corporatewide training session for existing employees and incorporated the customer service standards into performance reviews at all levels.

Corporatewide Training

Long-term employees have some of their own unique training needs. Because old habits die hard, this group may have to experience a paradigm shift to get in sync with the now-stated core values and customer service standards. This group will need to see proof that things are going to change. If 20 years

Figure 6-5. New-Employee Customer Service Orientation Outline

Supplies needed:

Flip chart
Customer service standard cards
Video: *Customer Service in Healthcare*

1. Welcome to WMH. Introduce Self.

   Why customer service?
   Overhead 1—Quote from Harvard Associate Dean
   Overhead 2—Ladder representing the levels of marketing results
   • People often think of advertising as the same thing as marketing.
   • Advertising really only influences the three bottom rungs on the ladder.
   • The real moment of truth comes when a patient or customer walks through the door. The encounter will ultimately determine the likelihood that they will return.
   • The ultimate in loyalty is positive word of mouth.

2. What do people expect from us? Excellence, skill, and care.

   Compare the level of expectation you have regarding a meal at a restaurant and health care.
   Health care is personal and emotional.

3. How do we know what our customers have to say about us?
   • Patient survey
   • Employee survey
   • Physician survey
   Overheads of quotes from surveys

4. Who are your customers?
   • List internal and external customers
   • Can you see how the needs and expectations of each of these groups may differ?

5. Customer service video

6. Hand out standards
   • Explain how standards were created and by whom.
   • Explain how they are used in evaluation process.
   • Ask them to sign as a commitment.

Questions or comments about standards

Welcome to our customer service team.

of complacency have been tolerated, why should they believe it will be any different now? If lousy performers have been rewarded with longevity, why should they believe things will change? Even more important than the initial training for this group will be the daily monitoring and feedback from the managers. In addition, this group will have to see evidence that management and administration are sincere about the standards through role modeling, recognition, and performance evaluations.

If "but we've always done it this way" has been the corporate theme song, stepping into a new, service-driven culture may be extremely difficult for employees who have been "raised" with a more lax set of expectations. Management's daily influence is the key to fostering change among existing employees.

Make Training Accessible and Diversified

Three shifts a day, 365 days a year make training a challenge for hospitals. In order to make sessions available to all employees, we held 12 sessions over several weeks and overlapped all shifts. The upside of this approach was that it made it easier for the patient care areas to send staff without leaving their departments short. The downside was the time demanded of the customer service team that conducted the training sessions. Each session was time away from the team members' regular jobs, which meant that their managers and coworkers had to be supportive of the initiative. We were very fortunate to have full support from the affected departments during the intensive training session.

Like the techniques used in the management education sessions, training sessions for the employees were designed to hold participants' attention and get them involved. In addition to lectures, we incorporated videos, discussion, role-play, and a self-assessment.

Our CEO opened each training session with a strong statement about the need for customer service excellence. Delivered in the context of our mission and vision, he asked each employee to accept the challenge of creating a place where patients want to be treated, where physicians want to practice, and where employees want to work.

With each group we made a special point of recognizing their fellow employees who had helped to design the standards. Seeing and hearing the names behind the product boosted credibility for the standards. Figure 6-6 outlines the format and agenda for the employee in-service training session. We allowed two hours for each session.

Who Should Be Included in the Training Sessions?

In addition to all employees within the organization, we included all volunteers and extended the invitation to all the medical staff and their office employees.

Our hospital, like most others, relies on the support of an active core of volunteers. These individuals are often the first faces our customers see when entering the building. They are a vital part of the hospital and, hence, the customers' experience. Including them in customer service training and orientation has proven a very worthwhile endeavor. The volunteers feel more valued when they are included in training sessions. And because of their volume and visibility, they have been an important part of the cultural shift toward service excellence.

We included the active medical staff and their clinic employees for several reasons. First and foremost, the patient experience often begins in the clinic setting. If we lose the customer there, we will never have them as patients in the hospital or outpatient services. The second reason is that even though we are separate businesses, the patients see us as one medical community. They rarely separate their doctor and staff from the hospital. This may not be the case in larger metropolitan areas, but for us it is a reality. And, finally, we included the clinic staffs because it helps to build collegiality between the organizations.

The majority of our medical staff sent their entire personnel. In fact, several of them made it mandatory. The feedback

Figure 6-6. Customer Service Team's Employee In-Service Training Format and Agenda

Customer Service Team: Dot Steinhorst, Mary Morstad, Laverne Schauer, Kris Baird, Janet Triplett, Linda Surdick, Steve Dana, Julie Albright, Sandy Roberts, Kathy Moody, Kathy Wolff

Goal: To provide a clear and consistent overview of customer service (CS) expectations to all WMH employees.

Objectives: Participating employees will:

- Be able to recognize categories and needs of customers
- Understand customer service standards and corporatewide expectations
- Understand personal accountability for performing according to established CS standards
- Understand consequences for noncompliance with the established CS standards
- Recognize their own unique personality traits and how they influence their ability to relate to others
- Discuss tools for dealing with difficult interpersonal situations

Format and Agenda for Employee Training

Objective Being Addressed	By Whom	Outline of Subject Discussed	Method Used	Est. Time
• Corporatewide expectations • Personal accountability	John K.	Why customer service? What we expect of you How CS pertains to your review	Lecture	10 min.
• Recognize categories and needs of customers	Kris B.	Why customer service? Who are your customers? List How many of you provide good CS? If we are providing good service, how do these things happen here? • Way finding • Confidentiality and talking over patient in elevator • Telephone—first impression • Respect	Discussion Role-play	10 min. 20 min.

(Continued on next page)

Figure 6-6. (Continued)

Objective Being Addressed	By Whom	Outline of Subject Discussed	Method Used	Est. Time
• Understand customer service standards	Kris	Explain how standards were created and by whom.	Lecture	5 min.
	Focus group members	Pass out cards and talk about standards.	Discussion, read	15 min.
• All	Jan	*Customer Service* video	Video	15 min.
Break				10 min.
• Understand customer ser- vice standards and corporate- wide expectations • Understand personal accountability for performing according to established CS standards	Focus group members	Coworkers are your customers too. Standards aren't just for external customers. Holding each other accountable	Lecture and discussion	15 min.
• Tools for deal- ing with difficult inter- personal situations	Dr. Duffin	Techniques for dealing with difficult coworkers	Discussion	15 min.
• Recognize their own unique personality traits and how they influence their ability to relate to others • Discuss tools for dealing with difficult inter- personal situations	Jan	Do personality traits assessment. Discuss how personality traits influence how you interact with others and how people see you.	Write Discussion	5 min. 15 min.
All	Kris	Summary of session including where do we go from here? Department action plans	Lecture	5 min.
All		Evaluation	Written	5 min.
		Respect video	Video	8 min.

we received from the physicians and staff was overwhelmingly positive. They not only had fun but felt they learned very useful techniques. A sample invitation to medical staff is shown in figure 6-7.

Session Evaluations

After each session, employees were asked to complete an evaluation (figure 6-8). The evaluations were designed to critique the training sessions as well as to identify attitudes, perceptions,

Figure 6-7. Invitation to Medical Staff

Dear Members of the WMH Medical Staff,

Excellent customer service has never been more important. As health care competition heats up, providers will be judged not only on medical outcomes, but on patient satisfaction as well. A unified, consistent approach to customer service training for all of our employees is one way we can ensure that Watertown providers will stand out from our competitors.

For the past several months, the WMH customer service team has been developing a comprehensive employee training program designed to enhance customer relations. The team will be holding several training sessions over the next two months and would like to extend this training opportunity to you and your staff.

Enclosed you will find a list of the dates, times, and locations for the training sessions. In order to accommodate all employees and volunteers, we will be accepting registrations on a first-come first-serve basis. If you and your employees would like to participate in the training, please indicate your session choice(s) on the attached form and forward to _____ in human resources. We will confirm these registrations as soon as we have matched the requests with available space.

We look forward to working with you and your staff on this vital initiative. Thank you in advance for your interest.

Sincerely,

Kris Baird
VP Business Development and Marketing

Figure 6-8. Customer Service Training Program's Participant Survey

---

Tell us what you think!

About the customer service training program

Please rate the following:

	Poor	Fair	Average	Good	Excellent
How well the objectives were met	O	O	O	O	O
Variety of teaching/learning techniques	O	O	O	O	O
How well the program held your interest	O	O	O	O	O
Clarity of customer service standards	O	O	O	O	O

About the videos and exercises

Please rate the following on how well they helped to meet the objectives:

	Poor	Fair	Average	Good	Excellent
Customer Service video	O	O	O	O	O
Coworker video	O	O	O	O	O
Assessment of personality traits (written)	O	O	O	O	O
Role playing	O	O	O	O	O
Respect video	O	O	O	O	O

As a result of this program, do you feel WMH employees will:

Have a clearer understanding of internal and external customers?   Yes   No

Have a clear understanding of the standards?   Yes   No

Do you feel the standards created are reasonable and attainable?   Yes   No

Who could you contact if you felt a coworker was not acting according to the established standards?_____

General attitudes about customer service at WMH

1. After participating in this training session, how likely are you to act in accordance with the standards presented?

very unlikely   somewhat unlikely   neither   somewhat likely   very likely

2. How confident are you that WMH will improve its customer service as a result of this hospitalwide training initiative?

very confident   somewhat confident   neither   somewhat uncertain   very skeptical

3. What else is needed to improve customer service at WMH?

4. What else can we do to improve this training program?

and any misgivings about the customer service initiative. The evaluations helped us immediately to make modifications where indicated. Skepticism about administration's commitment to enforcing the standards was evident, and this information helped us to understand our role even more clearly. We learned that we had to continually keep the customer service information in front of managers for daily reinforcement.

Graduating to a Second-Generation Customer Service Team

Now that the training sessions are over, it is a good time to breathe new life into the customer service team by bringing new members onto the team and relieving some of the long-term members of their duties. Preparation for this transition could actually begin months in advance as the team develops the training sessions. The customer service champion can prepare team members by telling them that their term will end after the training sessions in order to bring others on board in the customer service effort.

Creating a new team following the training sessions serves two purposes. First, it gives relief to the team members who have been working for months to roll out the training sessions. Second, it is an ideal time to recruit new members who have been inspired by the training sessions.

Summary

The training sessions are your chance to get everyone within the organization on the same page. Reading about the training and planning an outline are one thing. But delivering the message with passion and conviction is quite another. In order to be successful, the training sessions must be fun, accessible, informational, and believable. However, after months of preparation the training sessions can give a false sense of culmination. The reality is that they merely set the stage for the initiative.

The real work begins in keeping the effort alive and well and at the core of daily activity. The next chapter offers techniques that will help to keep the standards at the heart of daily activity.

References

1. Marsha Borling, "Improving Customer Service? Start at the Top," *Spectrum* (March/April 1998): 8–9.

2. Marsha Borling, owner, Borling and Associates, Gurnee, IL, interview with author, Chicago (May 14, 1998).

CHAPTER SEVEN

Keeping the Effort Alive

Objectives

After completing this chapter the reader will:

- Recognize the importance of keeping customer service in the forefront of daily operations long after the initial training is over

- Have strategies and tactics for maintaining top-of-mind awareness of customer service among employees

Keeping the customer service effort alive requires an understanding of what motivates people and a recognition that there are different learning styles. In chapter 6 we demonstrated that learning needs vary with longevity, job requirements, and responsibility. This chapter addresses the many methods available for keeping customer service at the forefront in your organization. Bear in mind that everyone learns through different methods. Some are readers, some are listeners, and some are doers. Educators categorize these classic learning styles as visual, auditory, and kinesthetic. But regardless of the terms used, the key message is that in order to keep the effort alive and at the core of your organizational culture, you need to understand and respect the different learning styles and plan to send the message in a variety of ways. In doing so, you greatly improve the odds that the message is getting through.

Encouraging a desirable culture takes consistent and persistent effort. It won't happen by default; it must be by design. Therefore, stating the mission and values once a year isn't enough to motivate behavior. Ask yourself how well your organization is formally communicating its customer service values. Are the values interwoven into the departments' regular staff meeting agendas as well as printed communications? Are they followed throughout the organization? Do they stop at the top leadership, or do they penetrate through to the front-line staff, volunteers, and medical staff?

This chapter offers proven tactics for weaving the core values throughout the organization consistently and by design. From printed communications to department meeting agendas, the message of service excellence must be consistently repeated, recognized, and rewarded in order to become the culture.

The Real Work Begins

After completing the training sessions, it may be tempting to breathe a sigh of relief with a sense of completion. While it's important to give yourselves a pat on the back, the real work is far from over. At this point, you have introduced the standards, completed the management and staff training, and reviewed the evaluation tools that will help measure and monitor staff performance in relation to customer service. But telling others what you expect is just the beginning. Until now, the staff and managers may have been passively listening to others talk about customer service, which won't bring it to life. In fact, chances are quite good that the employees have already classified the training sessions as the hospital's or clinic's "flavor of the month." They've seen programs come and go like the seasons, and in their minds this one is no different.

A culture shift takes time and persistence, but most of all it requires a series of experiences that will demonstrate that there is validity to the words that have been spoken. Try as you may, you cannot simply announce to employees on Monday, "Attention everyone, we're going to have a culture change. We want our customers to be thrilled with us and loyal to us for life. You are in charge of making sure this goal is reached. Please have your minds, attitudes, and hearts shifted to the new standards by Friday. Thank you and have a nice day."

Besides stating your expectations for customer service, you must demonstrate their value and recognize top performers regularly. Several strategies and tactics can help you to achieve this goal.

Departmental Action Plans

At the end of the management training session at Watertown, we presented a format for a departmental action plan. Each manager was to facilitate departmental meetings where staff would identify their customers and customers' core concerns and needs and set goals to meet the defined needs. Recognizing that many of the managers were already working at full capacity, we recommended that each manager appoint a lead person within his or her department to help coordinate the department meetings and prepare the final plan.

In addition to preparing a template for managers to follow, as presented in figure 6-4 in chapter 6, we offered them a prepared agenda for conducting the initial staff meeting. We also asked that they show a 16-minute video on coworker relations during this meeting.[1] Showing the video would help to reiterate and reinforce some of the messages heard during the original staff training. Our goal was to help managers organize the planning process with as little hassle as possible. We did stress, however, that they were free to follow their own process as long as the end result was a plan that encompassed the following:

- Identification of customer groups
- Determination of customer groups' core needs
- Assessment of the department's current ability to meet the customer needs
- Proposed actions to improve customer service
- Preparation of a method for measuring results

From an administrative perspective, I wanted to let the managers know that we were serious about the customer service initiative. Serious enough to hold them accountable for action plans. But we also wanted to communicate that we understood that they couldn't do it alone. Each manager in every department had to build buy-in among their subordinates. By collaborating with staff members in the creation of the action plan, managers were sending the message that "we're in this together."

We also let the managers know that as a department, the administrative team would be preparing an action plan as well.

The administrative team and department managers reconvened after one month to share their action plans. The depth and quality of the plans varied significantly. In hindsight, I would have had the managers share their plans with their administrative supervisor prior to the group meeting. That way, the administrator could have helped the manager to refine the plans where indicated.

Putting the plans into action is significantly harder than putting them on paper. Each manager had to define how the plans would be put into place and how to measure the results.

Checking plan progress became a shared responsibility for the administrative, supervisory, management, and department staff. I recommend quarterly reports as a means of keeping the plans in action. This keeps the effort "top-of-mind" and as vital as budget reports.

Make Your Promise Visible

Making a promise, then putting it in print brings it to a new level of sincerity. By placing our standards throughout the building, we were taking an intention and making it into a pledge. Since our standards were divided into internal and external subgroups, we made two sets of plaques that hang throughout our hospital and clinics. Both include the hospital mission statement and outline our commitment to service.

"Our pledge to you" plaques (figure 7-1) hang in every area where the patients and public go. "Our pledge to one another" (figure 5-1 in chapter 5) hangs in offices, nurses' stations, and meeting rooms where staff congregate. Both provide visual reminders to all of us about our promise.

We also made the plaques available to the medical office personnel who participated in our customer service training sessions. Several area physicians requested plaques for waiting rooms and employee break rooms. By extending the pledge to other medical practices associated with our hospital, we are building continuity.

Provide Patient Satisfaction Data

In order to maintain a level of enthusiasm for customer service plans, it's important to show departments that their efforts are making a difference. Every quarter, managers throughout our organization receive patient satisfaction data reports and are expected to share and interpret the data with their staff.

Figure 7-1. Pledge to External Customers

External Customers: Our pledge to you (patients and visitors)

"Welcome me."

Customer need: The need to feel welcome. *Our response:* We will reach out and be friendly.

- We will welcome you with a smile.
- We will state our names and use yours when available.
- If we're unsure of your needs we will ask if you need help.
- We will walk you to your destinations rather than giving verbal instructions.

"Comfort me."

Customer need: The need for comfort. *Our response:* We will handle you with care.

- We will protect your privacy and dignity by knocking before entering a room and not discussing private matters in public.
- We will solve problems within our authority. If we can't solve it, we'll find someone who can.
- We will respond quickly, and we'll explain delays.
- We will keep your surroundings as pleasant as possible, including keeping noise to a minimum.

"Understand me and help me understand."

Customer need: The need to understand and be understood. *Our response:* We will keep you informed.

- We will take the time to listen and give you our full attention.
- We will make explanations brief and easy to understand by using language you can understand.
- We will make sure you have the information you need.
- We will explain what we are doing and why we are doing it.

"Respect me."

Customer need: The need to be treated with respect. *Our response:* We will talk *to* you, not *at* you.

- We will include you in our conversations.
- We will be attentive, genuine, and positive.
- We will take the time to be courteous and considerate.
- We will involve you in decisions that concern your care.

Customer
Service
Standards

My pledge to WMH

**Watertown Memorial
Hospital**

Departments are invited to request more information, including cross-tab correlation between variables. To help facilitate managers' analysis of the data, we send out quarterly feedback forms (figure 7-2). Managers use this form to identify trends in the data and request more information from our quality resources department. It also serves as a reminder to pass the information along to department staff.

Coach the Coaches

Managing and coaching require two very distinct sets of skills. Although management skills are important to a smooth operation, coaching skills are probably more vital in creating and fostering a culture of service excellence. Management experts agree that coaching is a learned skill, not one with which you are born. If an organization wants to rise to a level of service excellence, there needs to be a plan for developing coaching skills. Following are a few suggestions to help improve coaching and leadership skills among managers:

- Work with human resources on a management education plan that offers ongoing training and reinforcement of coaching and leadership skills.
- Get the administrative team involved in creating a most valuable coach award on a quarterly basis. Be certain to correlate the award to the data and standards.
- Identify core leadership standards for managers to follow. Tie leadership standards to measurable goals and annual visionary leadership awards.
- Keep customer service "front and center" with staff.

Communication

Customer service values can be disseminated in a number of ways, including employee newsletters, bulletin boards, and special events.

**Figure 7-2. Quarterly Manager Review of Patient
Satisfaction Data**

Manager/coordinator _____ Unit _____

Data quarter _____

What trends have you identified?

1.

2.

3.

4.

5.

Are there any significant issues you would like to investigate further?
Y N If so, what?

What (if any) action plans is your department taking in order to improve
services?

What additional data would you like to investigate in order to facilitate
improvement? (Kris Baird or Kathy Moody can help to identify and
retrieve supporting data from database.)

How has this information been shared with your department?

Please return this form to Kris Baird, VP Business Development.
Thank you.

Employee Newsletters

Employee newsletters provide a natural vehicle for regular reminders about customer service expectations. Our CEO writes a message in every newsletter that ties mission and values to strategies and actions. Several messages each year pertain to customer service and its relationship to mission.

If your organization has an in-house newsletter, use it as a vehicle to continually keep employees up-to-date on customer satisfaction scores and comments. Be aware that many of the comments will be focused on employees involved in direct patient care, so you will have to identify ways to draw out feedback about the non-patient care areas as well. We solved this issue by publishing a coupon every month that could be clipped and passed from one employee to another as a means of recognizing extra effort. (See the section on coupons below.)

Our hospital makes a point of printing positive patient comments in the monthly newsletter and ties them back to the customer service standards. In addition to the patient comments, we print suggestions from employees about how to make our customers feel more welcome. These comments are gathered monthly at an Annual Education Day. In addition to focusing on the safety drills and updating staff on Joint Commission regulations, we use the Annual Education Day to gather employees' input on how to make Watertown Area Health Services a more customer-friendly environment.

We publish a column entitled "Notable Names" in the employee newsletter and cite patient and employee comments about stellar customer service.

Bulletin Boards

Keeping customers at the center of our actions requires keeping their feedback at the center of our attention as well. If we limit customer satisfaction reports to quarterly summaries only, the data are old and cumbersome. Having bulletin boards in every department with current satisfaction scores will help keep the initiative alive and real for everyone. If you set goals to improve service but don't show the team how it is doing, it's like players not knowing what yard line they are on in football. Department bulletin boards are a great way to get staff involved in motivating and encouraging teammates.

Annual Education Day

Our organization requires annual review of safety policies and procedures. In order to streamline the complexities involved in executing retraining, we offer an Annual Education Day. The same program is held once every month to accommodate employees' schedules and avoid a staffing drain on the departments. In addition to reviewing safety policies and procedures, we include a section on customer service.

Employees review the standards and identify positive and negative experiences with customer service. Figure 7-3 outlines our customer service discussion during the Annual Education Day in 1998. Figure 7-4 outlines an exercise we developed for 1999. Participants complete the exercise and seal it in an envelope with their name and department. We mail it back in three months for them to reevaluate their progress toward their personal goals.

Recognize, Reinforce, and Reward

See the behavior and praise it. It's as simple as that. I recently held a series of employee focus groups in which I was attempting to identify employee attitudes about rewards and recognition programs. The overriding opinion was that programs are not nearly as valuable to employees as a word of recognition from their immediate supervisors. Employees felt that because many of their managers didn't comment on their performance or thank them for extra effort, their actions were not appreciated. Verbal recognition is free and can be habit-forming. Not

Figure 7-3. Annual Education Day Team Discussion Outline

Each team should expand on one example in each of the following categories.

1. Worst customer service experiences outside of health care. Describe situation and how you felt.

   What made it a bad experience?

   What could have made the bad situation better?

2. Describe an example of some of the best customer service you've witnessed outside of health care (shopping, restaurants, telephone interactions).

   Describe situation and how you felt.

   What made it a good experience?

3. Describe one of the worst customer service experiences within a health care setting. Describe the situation and how you felt.

   What made it a bad experience?

   What could have made the bad situation better?

   How could you have let the person providing the service know that he or she had done an insufficient job?

4. Describe one of the best customer service experiences you've seen *within a health care setting.* Describe the situation and how you felt.

   What made it a good experience?

   How could you (or did you) let the person providing that service know that he or she had done a good job?

What can we do at WAHS to make our customers feel more welcome?

Figure 7-4. Identifying Customers and Their Needs

1. From the list below, *circle* the three customer groups with whom you have the most contact on a regular basis.
2. In the second column, next to the customer group you have just circled, list the things that customer needs or expects from you.
3. Now, imagine that you have to grade yourself on how well you currently meet those customer needs (at least 90 percent of the time). In the last column, give yourself a letter grade (A-B-C-D-F).

Customer Group	Customer Needs	Your Grade
Patients		
Coworkers		
Physicians		
Families/visitors		
Businesses		
Vendors		
Volunteers		
Others		

List 2 to 3 things that you (personally) will do to improve customer service.

1. _____
2. _____
3. _____

List something that you can do immediately to make your department a better place to work. _____

only can your organization benefit from managers' recognizing their subordinates, but also you will see employee morale climb when coworkers learn to recognize one another.

I'll never forget a simple lesson learned from a child's perspective about the importance of reinforcing positive behaviors. My three daughters and I were about to leave the house one morning. Harried as usual, I was trying to hustle all three girls, backpacks, briefcase, and lunches out the door to get to school, day care, and work on time. In the final dash to the car, three-year-old Hillary stopped to pick up some trash that had blown from the neighbor's garbage can. Without saying a word, she gathered it up from our sidewalk and deposited it in the garbage, then proceeded to climb into her car seat.

Five-year-old Lesley clapped and said, "Hillary, you are such a good citizen. You picked up that litter without even being told. Mom, isn't she a good citizen?"

Judging by Hillary's reaction, I knew that this would not be the last time she took the initiative to tidy up the yard. Not only did she get a round of applause and kind words from her older sister (an authority figure), the commendation was passed along to mom (the CEO of domestic affairs).

This simple lesson on reinforcing positive behaviors made a lasting impression. I learned that immediate recognition and reinforcement of good behavior, even from peers, can help shape our environment. If every employee would take the extra initiative to make the workplace a little cleaner, a little happier, we'd all enjoy our work more.

Reinforcing good behavior can't just happen between management and line staff. It has to become part of the culture.

Coupons and Prizes

Recognition for a job well done is often more gratifying than money. Companies all over the world have incentive programs and goals for performance. One low-cost incentive for customer service is based on coworkers' recognizing one another's outstanding customer service behavior. An easy way to accomplish this is to give employees access to coupons that they fill out and present to a coworker, identifying a customer service behavior that the individual demonstrated above and beyond the normal course of duty. The coupon recipient presents the coupon for a small token prize such as candy, water bottles, or mugs. The coupon is then entered into a monthly drawing for cash prizes.

One organization holds the drawing in the cafeteria the first Monday of the month. All employees are invited to witness the drawing conducted by the CEO. The CEO uses the drawing as a forum to thank the staff for their customer service efforts and to remind them of their importance to the mission and vision. He draws the winning coupons and reads the comments that describe the customer service action and the name of the recipient. This form of public recognition can go a long way in keeping efforts alive.

Public Praise

Publicly praising employees for stellar performance reinforces the behavior with peers. One hospital in Florida has a "Notable Names" banner in the hospital cafeteria. When specific employees are named on surveys for customer service, they get to sign their names on the banner. In their organization, it is quite prestigious to be included on the banner.

Holy Cross Hospital in Chicago spotlights its "Value Stars" every month on a lobby marquee. Peers or patients nominate employees for exemplary performance of one or more of the hospital's core values. Their stories are shared publicly at a recognition dinner.

Formal Recognition Programs

There are numerous ways organizations can recognize employees for outstanding performance. The options are almost endless.

But in order to keep customer service at the core of the recognition program, you must tie the standards back to performance and measurable goals. There should be opportunities for team, as well as individual, awards. Team awards can be tied to patient satisfaction scores on the nursing units, for example. Individual awards can be implemented with a system like the ones mentioned above. But regardless of the actual method used, to gain credibility and visibility the rewards should be clearly linked to the stated core values and customer service standards.

Cues to Signal One Another

Some organizations have been very successful at developing verbal and nonverbal signals to let workers know how they are doing. One hospital staff developed a phrase that would signal a coworker that he or she was behaving outside the acceptable standards. When someone observed negative behavior in front of patients or other staff, they simply said, "That's off track." To share a compliment, they would say, "That was really on track." These signals can help make workers more aware of their actions and allow them to correct them on the spot.

Another organization stressed its goal of providing "WOW" service rather than "bow-wow" service. Employees were given laminated dog bones. If they observed a fellow employee being rude or abrupt, they would quietly pass him or her a bone to show that the behavior was out of line with expectations.

Hiring for Optimal Customer Service

In previous chapters I emphasized the importance of hiring for customer service. The magnitude of this step in the scope of the overall culture makes it worthy of repetition. To keep the effort alive, you must hire only people who will live by the standards. This may require coaching and mentoring managers to spot desirable characteristics in candidates.

All the incentive programs in the world won't build a customer-focused environment without the right people in place. Many organizations place a high value on personality profiles, such as the Meyer's Briggs test, to determine whether a job candidate will fit into the team. Other organizations have their own set of assessments that zero in on personality traits. Still others settle for résumés and hope for the best.

If your organization doesn't have a formal mechanism for assessing candidates, it may be worthwhile to look at other companies that have successfully implemented applicant-screening programs.

Summary

Keeping customer service efforts alive in your organization doesn't have to be costly or complicated. It does, however, have to be consistent in order to foster the cultural change. Once you have completed the customer service training sessions, you will need to keep the standards in front of the staff. The second-generation customer service team can spearhead programs such as the ones identified in this chapter. But regardless of who actually implements the actions, the rewards and recognition must be linked back to the standards and core values in order to remain credible.

Reference

1. *Positive Co-worker Relations in Healthcare,* video (LaCrosse, WI: Health-care Video Productions, 1990).

CHAPTER EIGHT

Customer Service Pointers for Physicians

Objectives

After completing this chapter the reader will:

- Recognize the importance of customer service in physician practice development

- Appreciate the importance of patient perception in predicting loyalty

- Learn communication techniques to enhance patient relations

- Be able to identify customer groups, including patients

This chapter is written expressly for physicians in an attempt to address the customer service challenges specific to the medical profession. First, allow me to give my disclaimer. The term *customer* is used throughout this chapter because it represents several groups including, but not limited to, patients. I have encountered more objections from physicians about the term *customer* than I care to count. For logical reasons, physicians resent their patients being referred to as customers. There are times when it is perfectly appropriate to segregate the patients from the rest of the customer subgroups, particularly when referring to them specifically. I do, however, want to impress upon the physician reader that there are several other groups of individuals who, through their direct and indirect contact with you and your practice, will form opinions that have a bearing on your professional and financial success. They have not yet stepped into an exam room or shared a medical history with you, but they have formed opinions about you and your practice. Furthermore, these individuals can and will express their opinions about you to others. They are the parents, caretakers, drivers, friends of patients, mail carriers, hospital nurses, or vendors who come in contact with you and your clinic staff. Your staff and physician peers are two additional groups of customers who can, and do, influence your business every day.

To prove my point, just take a look around the waiting room. At almost any time during the day individuals other than patients will be occupying the waiting room. They are listening to the receptionist, observing patients' wait time, watching physician/staff interaction, and ultimately forming opinions about what they observe. It takes approximately 30 seconds to form an opinion. Most of your nonpatient customers will have closer to 30 minutes to observe and judge your practice during an average contact.

Although I recognize that using the word *customer* may raise physicians' ire, I would be remiss to imply that patients are the only group of people who can have an impact on your business.

What Customer Service Means to Your Bottom Line

In the face of rising managed care and shrinking reimbursement, it doesn't take a rocket scientist to understand the need for increased patient volume. And the biggest impact you can make on volume begins with retaining your existing customers. Consider these facts:

- It is 6 to 10 times more costly to attract a new customer than it is to retain an existing one.
- Ninety-six percent of your unhappy customers will never complain to you. They are, however, talking to friends, family, coworkers, and others. In fact, on average, a dissatisfied patient will tell approximately 20 other people.
- As many as 90 percent of unhappy customers will quietly seek another provider without your ever hearing from them.
- Satisfied patients will tell only 5 other people.
- When one patient/customer complains to you, there are 15 others sitting silently behind him or her. In other words, only one in 15 will actually speak up.

Perception Is Reality

Referring to patient concerns, I can't tell you how many times I have heard physicians say, "That's just their perception." The hard truth is that a patient's perception is that patient's reality. Patients' perceptions will lead them to speak positively or negatively about your medical practice. Their perceptions may lead to multiple referrals or countless missed opportunities. If you don't think perceptions are reality, consider the last time that you had a less-than-desirable dining experience. Chances are you left saying, "I'll never go there again." Your decision was based on perceptions of service, quality, courtesy, and atmosphere. It wouldn't matter to you if the restaurant rated five stars in the dining guide—your own perception would dictate your loyalty. Your patients are no different. While your degrees and certificates may be an initial attraction for new patients, if they perceive less-than-excellent service, chances are they will not return. And they will tell up to 20 others.

In his book *Patients Build Your Practice,* Michael Cafferky cites the following statistics. "As many as 95 percent of all unhappy people will not tell a doctor that they are unhappy with the service they received. However, they are willing to tell someone else. In fact, marketing experts say that people who are unhappy with a doctor's service are 10 times more likely to speak about their unhappiness to someone else than is someone who is happy with the service received."[1]

You may feel that you have excellent rapport with your patients. You may be perfectly comfortable with your communication style, diagnostic capabilities, and bedside manner. But patient perceptions aren't formed by your relationship alone. Cafferky states: "Up to 80 percent of lost clients can be attributed to a problem with the people who work at a practice. It might be indifference, poor performance, or just lack of the ability to get along with people."[2]

When collecting data for my master's thesis, I had the opportunity to survey patients from 17 area clinics regarding their perception of the quality of care. It was no surprise that their perceptions of quality had little to do with the physician's competence, diagnostic abilities, or clinical outcomes. In fact, it had little to do with whether they felt better as a result of their visit. The key factors influencing their perceptions of quality in the clinic setting had to do with the human elements. Did they feel listened to? Did they have to wait long to get an appointment? Did the doctor or nurse explain their condition and treatments to them? Here are some of the common comments made:

- "I couldn't get in when I wanted."
- "The 'nurse' was rude on the phone" (consumers often refer to all females in clinics as nurses).

- "They don't even look up when I come into the office. I feel like I'm interrupting them."
- "The first question is always 'what insurance do you have?' not 'how can we help you?'"
- "The only time the receptionist smiles is when she is asking for my co-pay."
- "If I want to talk to the doctor, the staff makes me feel like I'm going through national security checks."
- "I was transferred so many times that I just hung up."
- "They put me in an exam room and just forgot me."
- "No one explained anything to me. I went home more confused than when I came in."

Before you dismiss these comments as "other people's problems" or insist that these things don't happen in your clinic, ask yourself the following questions:

- How do you know problems aren't happening here? Are you surveying your patients? Are you asking patients for their opinions during their office visits?
- Are you aware of whether the schedulers and receptionists are polite to callers?
- Do you routinely walk through the front door and sit in the waiting room to observe what your patients see?
- Have you clarified your expectations about service to your staff? And are you modeling the desirable behavior?

Being a good clinician isn't enough any more. The world has changed, and patients have come to expect a higher level of customer service. Like it or not, physicians and health care organizations are up against the Hiltons, Nordstroms, and Disneys of the world. These stellar organizations have raised the bar on customer service and shown the world that it is not only possible to deliver superb customer service, it's absolutely essential.

When customers choose a physician or a health care organization based on quality, they are actually choosing based on what is most real to them—service. How can they judge based on anything else? The customer, unless a medical professional, cannot possibly judge you as your peers would. Patients aren't conducting a utilization review or benchmarking best practices. They can, however, tell you how they have been served. And they will share their perceptions with others.

Consider the case of the pharmaceutical sales representative who demonstrates the influence she has on new referrals. I was at a baby shower for "Linda" and asked her how she had selected her physician. "For me it was easy," Linda said. "With all the visits I make to clinics in the area, I just watched how well the patients were treated and how well the physician interacted with the staff. I felt that physicians who were rude to me as a sales rep would probably be just as rude to me if I were a patient. Believe me, I know who's got the best credentials, and they aren't always someone I would have for my doctor. The same goes for the office staff. My waiting time in the clinics was a great chance for me to see how things really work. Some of the receptionists were so rude that I wouldn't ever go there as a patient."

Never underestimate the power of observation. Just as your observations lead to a more timely and accurate diagnosis, everyone coming in contact with you and your practice are making observations that lead to final decisions. Like you, they are picking up on the subtleties that reflect on your people skills.

A colleague of mine is a clinic manager. Troubled by the way one of the staff physicians interacted with his office personnel, "Carol" confided that one of the physicians had a reputation for reprimanding or even ridiculing his staff—often in front of patients. When Carol addressed this concern with the doctor, he denied that it was a problem, even though he had had a 400 percent turnover in front office staff in 18 months. He didn't take his conduct seriously until a patient said, "You're awfully hard on your staff; I'll bet they're looking forward to your vacation." At that point he realized that others were not only observing his behavior, but were forming negative opinions of him based on those observations.

Lip Service Just Won't Cut It with Your Staff

Setting clear expectations for your staff about customer service is essential. But it's even more important that you model behavior consistent with those stated expectations. For example, if you tell the staff that you expect patients to be seen within 20 minutes of their arrival but you don't return from lunch on time, you are setting the example that you aren't really serious about the rules. And you are setting them up for failure. After all, how can they meet the 20-minute goal if you aren't there?

The following principles, outlined for managers in previous chapters, can be applied in the clinic situation as well:

- Begin by hiring the right people for the job. That means looking beyond the degrees and certificates to the personality traits, values, and beliefs.
- Clarify your expectations to potential employees at the time of the initial interview and continue throughout their employment.
- Monitor and measure performance.
- Coach and manage performance through role modeling, rewards, and recognition.
- Develop customer-focused policies and procedures.

I have had numerous opportunities to launch new programs, clinics, and services from the ground floor up. In these situations it has been a challenge to bring a new group together and develop a mission, vision, and philosophy. The greatest advantage, however, was that we all started at the same point with the unique opportunity to create the environment that we felt would be the best for our patients and us. It is far more difficult to alter an existing culture, particularly one that is divergent from your core values.

Taking Small, Consistent Steps

In chapters 2 and 3 I addressed the importance of setting the stage for customer service very early in your relationship with your employees. If you haven't done so already, create a mission statement with your partners and office staff. In doing so, you are setting the stage for clear and consistent service. Not everyone buys into the need for a mission statement. But think of it this way—your mission statement is a reflection of your beliefs. It's a snapshot of who you are and what you stand for. It gives your patients, staff, and coworkers a sense of your deeper values and exposes a side of you that others may not see.

A mission statement can be a cluster of words on paper or a guiding force for your organization. The choice is yours. I firmly believe that companies that can state their missions clearly and concisely have a much better chance of coming out on top in a competitive environment. A mission sets the stage for individual and team performance if you are committed to it. It serves as a screening device to determine if you are on the right track and helps others to know what you stand for. Steven Covey recommends that each of us craft a mission statement for ourselves based on core values. The process Covey defines for developing a mission statement is fairly straightforward and may help you to clarify what is most important to you.[3]

Begin constructing your mission statement by involving your partners and office staff in an open discussion, preferably in a relaxed setting. Discuss the following points:

- What business are we in?
- Who are we serving?
- How do we want to be known?

Rather than trying to "wordsmith" a final draft as a collective group, jot down the key ideas on an overhead transparency or flipchart. Have one person summarize the ideas into a paragraph consisting of two to four sentences and distribute the draft to the participants for feedback.

Once you have written the clinic or department mission statement, you are ready to move forward in developing customer service standards. This process is explained in chapter 5.

Are You a Patient Advocate?

Most physicians would answer this question with an unequivocal "yes, of course." After all, didn't you go to medical school to serve your patients? But knowledge of the science of medicine didn't necessarily prepare you for patient advocacy. In today's rapidly changing health care environment, patients are confused about who the decision makers are and how to get their questions answered. Payers are demanding increased productivity and cost containment from the providers. At the same time, patients expect high-quality service and professional competency while silently fearing that they won't be able to pay the medical bills.

Patient advocacy is connected to patient satisfaction. When questions are answered clearly and respectfully, patients are much more likely to view you, your staff, and the entire organization in a more positive light. As employers and other third-party payers negotiate for volume discounts and select preferred providers, they are involving patients in identifying providers with value-added services. The exceptional providers will be the ones that can help customers navigate the system by clarifying billing questions, providing clear information about services, and helping them to make informed decisions about their care. These are just a few of the crucial factors that will separate your practice from the pack.

In their book *Putting the Patient First,* Bob Richards and Jeanan Yasiri outline many of the steps that health care providers can take to become better patient advocates. They take a very consumer-focused approach to helping providers understand how the customer sees the practice and what can be done to facilitate a better relationship between the customer and the practice as a whole.[4]

In a conversation with Bob Richards, I asked his opinion about where physicians typically fall short in their role as patient advocates. He responded with the following:

> Patients want to trust their doctors more than anyone else in the health care system. By the time a disgruntled patient speaks up, [that patient has] had anywhere from one to twelve bad incidents. I can't stress enough that when a physician receives a patient complaint, it is a huge turning point in his or her relationship with that patient. If they [physicians] can view the complaint as an opportunity to get at the patients' perceptions, they can begin to reestablish trust. A complaint is a huge opportunity to spot areas for improvement. This is often very difficult because it's our nature to become defensive and angry when challenged.

Richards and Yasiri devote an entire chapter of their book to tackling the tendency to be defensive. The tools and training outlined in their book can be applied to anyone dealing with customers, but it is particularly useful for physicians as well as billing and reception professionals.

Richards stresses the need to be reasonable in dealing with customer complaints. He says:

> Retailers often say, "the customer is always right." Health care providers would be doing a disservice to the customer by saying that they are right all the time. A patient advocacy stance is simply this: The customer is always entitled to a courteous answer. Saying that [the customer is] always right isn't fair to the provider or responsive to the customer's needs. Because, quite often, what the customer needs is more information. If we simply say "you're right, we're sorry," we won't be helping the customer to understand the system well enough to make decisions in the future. Take, for instance, a customer who is angry about a bill. Don't just lower it because he is angry. Communicate why the charges are appropriate, then determine if an adjustment is warranted.[5]

Richards stresses the need to be fair, responsive, and consistent. In doing so you will be setting the groundwork for a better understanding of your service.

Customer Service and Risk Management

What does customer service have to do with risk management? More than you might think. Very simply stated, people rarely sue people whom they like.

In many cases, formal medical education prepares students to be scientists. You learn to assess, diagnose, treat, and evaluate the results of your efforts. But where in the standard medical school curriculum is there a course of study that prepares students for the human elements of medicine? One can argue that you either have a good personality or you don't. You're either likable or you're not. To some degree that may be true, but you can learn to communicate better with your patients and other customers. In doing so you could actually reduce the amount of staff turnover, patient attrition, and the likelihood of a lawsuit.

Research has shown that if patients perceive that their physician has listened to their concerns, they will be more likely to comply with the doctor's orders and will have a higher perception of their overall care. Following some seemingly simple practices can significantly alter patient perceptions about a physician and the quality of the interaction. Here are just a few:

- Follow up with the patient about the last visit. "The last time you were here, we were trying some new approaches for your allergies. How is the new medication working for you?" This lets patients know that you remember them specifically and care enough to ask about their progress.
- Sit down at some point during the visit. This sends a nonverbal message that you are here to stay for a while.
- Look patients in the eye. This tells them that they have your undivided attention and demonstrates that what they are telling you is important to you. If you must write notes, or type in the case of electronic medical records, tell the patient what you are doing. "What you are telling me is

important. I want to be sure to make a quick note about it. Do you mind if I write (type) while you're talking?"

- Validate what patients are saying by repeating key statements like: "Let me make sure I understand. So you feel the pain gets worse after walking?"
- Verbalize that you are listening with short responses: "Uh huh"; "I see"; or "Tell me more about that."
- Wash your hands in the exam room in front of the patient. This demonstrates that you are preparing for the exam and leaves no doubt about infection control.
- Ask open-ended questions when possible to avoid yes or no responses. This engages the patient in a conversation as opposed to a checklist of answers.
- Answer questions thoroughly and clearly. Verify that all a patient's questions have been answered. Again, try to avoid yes or no answers. Rather than asking, "Do you have any other questions?" ask, "What other questions can I answer for you?"
- Summarize what you covered during the visit. This can prevent patients from leaving and feeling "the doctor didn't do anything." No one wants to leave a doctor's office with the feeling that the visit wasted time and money. Consumers of modern medicine are looking for magic bullets to cure everything. Being told "it's just a virus" leaves many patients feeling that they came to you unnecessarily. Let them know what was done. "I'm glad you came in. Because when I see someone with a fever and sore throat like yours, I want to check for some serious problems. I have ruled out encephalitis and scarlet fever with some of the tests I did today. That's a really good sign." Telling the customer what you have done to rule out various conditions lets them know you have covered some very important assessments.
- Let them know very clearly what to do next. When possible, give self-care or follow-up instructions in writing. When people are feeling stressed, they retain less information. By

providing information in writing, they can review the material when they are in a more receptive frame of mind. Ideally, patients would receive a follow-up call from you our your staff within 24 hours of the visit.

- Let patients know what to expect from you next. "I will be calling you tonight to check on your progress" or "I will be calling you tomorrow with your lab results."
- Emphasize self-responsibility. "As your doctor, I can only do so much. I can diagnose and prescribe the correct treatment, but you have to be the one to take the medication as prescribed. You and I have to be partners in this."

Mastering these communication skills can have a major impact on your patient's perception of you and the quality of the visit. If practiced consistently, you have a much better chance of being perceived as a good listener, a compassionate caregiver, and a thorough practitioner. But remember that your staff is equally important in crafting the impressions and perceptions of your customers. Help them to understand the importance of being liked. Patients share some of the most intimate details of their lives within the four walls of your practice and are far more likely to remain loyal to providers who demonstrate respect and courtesy in addition to clinical competence.

Don't Forget Your Other Customers

Although the majority of this chapter has been devoted to the patient customer group, there are a few others that warrant some attention. Your peers or medical colleagues, for instance, are an important group of customers. So are nurses and other clinicians and caregivers.

Colleagues

Consider the orthopedic surgeon who is known for his skill with sports injuries. He gladly accepts referrals from a neighboring family practice group but never communicates back to the referring physician. Worse yet, he undermines the referring physician's initial diagnosis to the patient, creating enough doubt that the patient transfers to another primary care clinic.

Or how about the physician who, without clinical indication, deviates from the established clinical pathway in spite of objections from the other members of the multidisciplinary team. Refusal to work collaboratively can be costly as well as a threat to quality outcome.

As with any team, it takes a variety of players to help reach specific goals. A collegial medical staff that can collaborate through difficult issues will foster a healthy work environment. I have witnessed some incredible quality improvement initiatives as a result of physicians putting aside their egos for the common good. Doctors who have mastered the art of collaboration know that there is certainly a difference between collaboration and "covering up" others' errors.

Like your patients, your colleagues want your respect and support. They want your prompt attention and a listening ear. And, at the very least, they want courtesy.

Nurses

Nurses as customers? Sure. Like patients, nurses make observations of you and form opinions about your skill level and personality. Even though you are their customer, at times they become yours as well. Nurses are your eyes and ears when you can't be with your patients. They provide a strong link between you and your patients and can greatly influence your reputation. They are at the bedside making sure that your orders are carried out. Yet in spite of their value, they are often discounted and disrespected by the very physicians who rely on them the most. I can't name one nurse associate that hasn't been screamed at, sworn at, or even threatened by physicians at one time or another in her career. It's unfortunate that such behavior is ever tolerated at all. There are enough demands on the nursing profession today without emotional and verbal abuse from physicians. Your mood or your workload is never an excuse for discourteous behavior.

Demonstrating consistent, courteous behavior will greatly enhance your working relationship with the nursing staff and improve the quality of patient care as a result.

Here are a few suggestions for improving your working relationship with nurses.

- Learn the nurses' names and use them.
- Show common courtesy—"please," "thank you," and "I'm sorry" can go a long way.
- Let them know you appreciate their help.
- Show them respect and draw them into the team.
- Ask their opinion. After all, the nurses are with patients 24 hours a day. And remember, they can learn many things from you and your colleagues. Use encounters to help educate the nurses about new treatments and your unique approach to care.

Besides being a vital part of the health care team, nurses are often the source of numerous referrals. Ask any nurse how often friends, neighbors, and family members consult her for advice about physician selection. The answer might surprise you. Most nurses report countless encounters every year. And even when a nurse is certain of a physician's clinical competency, she won't speak highly of a doctor with a poor bedside manner.

Summary

Physicians who take the time to clarify mission and values will have a much greater chance of improving the behavior of their staff. But actions speak louder than words. In order to build strong and lasting relationships with patients, colleagues, and office staff, physicians must practice a consistent set of customer-focused behaviors. Courtesy, showing respect, and good communication skills are qualities that can shape the course of a physician's career. Practicing some of the skills outlined in this chapter is a good starting point on the road to better customer service.

References

1. Michael E. Cafferky, *Patients Build Your Practice* (New York: McGraw-Hill, Inc., 1994), p. 4.

2. Ibid.

3. Steven Covey, *Seven Habits of Highly Successful People* (New York: Simon & Schuster, 1989).

4. Bob Richards and Jeanan Yasiri, *Putting the Patient First* (Englewood, CO: Medical Group Management Association, 1997).

5. Bob Richards, patient advocate, Dean Clinic, Madison, WI, interview with author (June 1, 1998).

CHAPTER NINE

A Message for Nurses

Objectives

After completing this chapter the reader will:

- Recognize the unique role nurses play in health care

- Understand the importance of customer service in patient and public perceptions about health care

- Recognize that attitude and judgment influence the nurse-patient relationship

- Learn action steps that can influence perceptions in every customer encounter

Believe it or not, this chapter was the most difficult one for me to write. Being a registered nurse myself, one would think that addressing nurses would be second nature. It is in most cases. But when I start to address the core issues surrounding customer service in nursing, I feel that each statement has to be so carefully weighed and measured that it's sometimes difficult to cut right to the chase. My hesitation is based on more than 20 years' experience in dealing with other nurses in a variety of settings. One common overriding theme I have discovered is nurses' strong desire to be the patient advocate. In striving to achieve that goal, however, many nurses lose sight of their role on the health care team.

This chapter is written specifically for nurses and can be presented in a number of ways. The individual nurse can read it, or its contents can be presented as a nursing in-service. If the in-service approach is the one chosen, it can be organized by the customer service champion and presented by the nurses on the customer service team. I strongly recommend having nurses present the information because it lends credibility to the subject at hand. Nurses from the customer service team can recruit other stellar performers (nurses) to assist with role-playing and storytelling as part of the presentation. Find comments from the surveys that will shed light on patient perceptions of nurses, both good and bad. Ask the presenting nurses to share real-life examples of good and bad customer service given by nurses.

The Role of the Nurse in Influencing Patient Perceptions

Our profession was founded with a strong belief in treating the whole person and serving as the truest of patient advocates. I have always felt that we have the best of both worlds in health care. We have a broad-based education that allows us to perform the most high-tech care while maintaining a close, nurturing relationship with the patient and family. But like the medical profession, as nursing became more technical, we began to lose sight of the human elements that have made our profession unique. In today's demanding health care environment, there is always an element of urgency to treat, medicate, assess, report, and so on. The pace will probably never slow. The shift from fee-for-service reimbursement to prospective payment has forced fundamental changes in staffing and length of stay that place nurses in their most challenging role ever—to do more with less *and* to do it in less time. But with today's consumers, clinical prowess isn't enough. Consumers expect us to have the clinical expertise. They expect us to be the advocate. But what makes or breaks their opinion of the entire organization often goes directly back to the quality of the nurses' personal interaction.

Nurses play a crucial role in shaping patient perceptions of health care. You cannot separate nurses from the total health care experience. Nurses are the face and personality of the organization. Nurses are the response time. Nurses are the pain management. Nurses are the source of information. Nurses are the compassion and concern. When nurses disappoint patients in any one of these areas, the overall perception of the organization declines.

Our first challenge is to take back our place in health care where we, the nurses, are the truest of patient advocates. Our second, but most crucial, challenge is to move beyond the "ain't it awful" thinking and accept the hand dealt us by managed care. Being customer service–focused requires a positive attitude and unwavering consistency in basic human relations.

This chapter focuses on actions and behaviors that will improve customer perceptions of the nurse and, hence, the organization. While seemingly simplistic, following this basic set of guidelines will enhance your role as a team member and patient advocate. Beginning with patient relations and concluding with other customer groups, this chapter was designed to help nurses enhance customer service behavior that can improve the internal working environment and enhance patient perceptions. Previous chapters particularly useful to nurses covered customer service departmental action plans (chapters 6 and 7 and figure 6-4)—designed to identify key customers, their needs, plans for service improvement, and measures of success—and employee service pledges to internal and external customers (chapters 5 and 7 and figures 5-1 and 7-1).

Patients enter health care settings with a common set of expectations. They expect that the professionals with whom they come in contact will have educational and technical skills that prepared them for their current positions. They expect to be kept informed and treated with respect. They want prompt and consistent responses to their concerns. When these expectations are met, patients usually give the provider a satisfactory rating. When unmet, they leave feeling slighted, angry, and sometimes hostile.

A challenge for nurses as well as other direct care providers is moving from satisfactory encounters to exceptional encounters. The following suggestions are not necessarily new or profound, but when practiced consistently they can help to move your satisfaction scores from satisfactory or good to exceptional or great.

Communication—Make It GREAT!

Beginning with your initial greeting and continuing throughout the patient encounter, communication skills help to shape the relationship. Some of the pointers I have included are so basic that many readers will wonder why I felt a need to even mention them. The truth is, it's the basics that are most often overlooked, particularly when we are busy or harried. We make assumptions that leave big voids in communication. The acronym GREAT helps caregivers to remember some basic communication skills:

- Greet the patient by introducing yourself
- Recap previous treatments or encounters

- *E*xplain what to expect next
- *A*sk for questions
- *T*ell patients when they can expect you back

Use this simple acronym to develop GREAT communication skills. Similar to a newspaper reporter, your patients are going to want to know who, what, when, where, and why. This acronym helps you to cover the key points. Review the GREAT list every time you enter a patient's room.

Greet with an Introduction

In the initial greeting, address the patient by name, using the most formal title until otherwise indicated. If patients don't offer a first name, it is appropriate for you to ask how they prefer to be addressed. Tell them who you are, giving your name and position.

"Good morning, Ms. Jones. I am Kris Baird, an RN on this unit, and will be caring for you today until 3:00 this afternoon."

I cannot begin to count the number of times that I have heard patients say that caregivers never introduced themselves during a clinic appointment or an entire hospital stay. Let patients and families know who you are and how you fit into the care environment. Always wear a nametag to identify yourself as part of the organization. I had a personal experience that gave me new insight into the importance of introducing myself as the nurse.

During high school, I was hospitalized for severe dehydration following a bout of flu. Over the course of a five-day stay, countless people came and went from my room without ever telling me who they were, what they did, or how I could contact them for help. One of the anonymous individuals had been adamant that I tell someone any time I needed to get up. She never said why it was important. For all I knew, it was their method of tracking patient migration patterns. She never said whom I should tell either. So when I had to get up to go to the bathroom, I told the first person who came into the room. She smiled and said "OK" and left. After nearly fainting in the bathroom, the nurse found me clinging to the wall on my way back to bed. She angrily demanded to know why I hadn't told anyone. I learned later that the "someone" I told was a house-keeper. I had no way of knowing if she was a nurse, a house-keeper, or the chief of surgery. I had simply done what I was told to do. Security is another reason to always introduce your-self and explain your role. Consider the following story of a new mother in the OB unit.

My friend "Cheryl" had just given birth to her first baby, a beautiful, healthy baby girl. Cheryl had the baby rooming in and was enjoying the quiet bonding time. The baby was resting qui-etly, so Cheryl decided to freshen up in the bathroom. While in the bathroom Cheryl heard someone call to her through the closed door: "I'm taking the baby for a weight. I'll be right back." By the time she opened the bathroom door, the baby and who-ever belonged to the voice on the other side of the door were gone. Trying to convince herself that she'd seen too many movies on newborn abduction, Cheryl tried to quell her fears, waiting for the baby to be returned. After 10 minutes she put on her call light. After another 5 minutes the light was answered. After another 2 minutes her question was answered. The situation had been simple. The nurse had taken the baby back to the nursery to be weighed. While in the nursery, the pediatrician arrived and decided to keep the baby for an assessment. The nurse was just about to return the baby when Cheryl called. By not introduc-ing herself or explaining what to expect, the nurse had subjected Cheryl to 17 minutes of unnecessary anxiety.

In hindsight, both Cheryl and the nurse learned some important lessons. The nurse learned not to take introductions and explanations for granted. Cheryl learned to ask for more information when it wasn't readily offered. If the nurse had been more customer focused, she would have known how important it was to make direct contact with the patient before removing the baby from the room.

Recap Previous Encounters or Treatments

This builds rapport by letting patients know that you remember what has happened with them previously. Even if you don't remember, you can review the chart prior to entering the room. Example: "I see that you had some pain medication at 5, how has that been working for you?"

Explain What to Expect Next

It's no secret that patients frequently feel overwhelmed and out of control in health care settings. By explaining treatment plans, nurses can include patients in the care plan. "I just want to review what will be happening today. As you know, you are scheduled for a series of tests. The first one requires a bowel prep that we will begin shortly. Once you have completed the prep, you will be taken to radiology."

Ask for Questions

Ask patients what additional information they may need. By inviting questions, you will be helping to keep them informed and address concerns or fears. Solicit questions with an open-ended invitation rather than a direct question. Don't ask, "Do you have any questions?" Rather, ask, "What additional information can I give you?"

Tell Them When They Can Expect to See You Again

And stick to your word. Hospitals can be scary places for many people. If your patients know when to expect you back, they are less likely to rely on call lights. One Florida hospital found a simple but useful tool for communicating nurses' return time. Nurses in this hospital placed cardboard clock faces on the doors of every patient room. When the nurse would leave, she would tell the patient when she planned on returning.

Then, she would set the scheduled time of return on the "clock." Of course the nurse would also invite patients to put on their call lights if any concerns arose before the scheduled return time. They found that patients used their call lights significantly less and nurses reported that it helped them with time management.

Rating Your Performance—You Be the Judge

When trying to improve your personal performance, it is often helpful to imagine that you are the one completing the patient satisfaction surveys and that the questions are about your own performance. Would you give yourself an average rating? Or would you judge your performance to be of star quality? If you are not scoring an excellent rating, ask yourself what you need to do to improve. The following topics are all directly correlated to overall patient satisfaction. Each area is within the nurse's circle of influence. By evaluating yourself and striving for stellar performance in each of these areas, you will be greatly improving patients' perception of the entire experience with your organization.

Promptness

Trust is a basic human need and is never more essential than when you are relying on others for care. Being prompt in responding to patients' needs will help to build trust. Using the clock tool cited above could actually help you to improve your response time because it helps you to schedule your visits.

Empathy

Being empathetic and showing empathy are two very different things. One dictionary defines empathy as "understanding so intimate that the feelings, thoughts, and motives of one are readily comprehended by another." In other words, empathy is cognitive and emotional but not necessarily behavioral. Caregivers may feel empathy yet never show it. Almost anyone struggling with physical or emotional pain will find comfort in knowing that another human being understands. There are some basic actions that, when done with sincerity, will help to demonstrate empathy. They include:

- Active listening demonstrated by eye contact and verbal and nonverbal validation (nodding, saying "uh huh," and so forth). Verbal validation shows that you are listening and understanding, such as saying "that must be very difficult for you." Avoid saying things like "I understand" because if you have not lived the same experience, you may not really understand.
- Touch—When appropriate, a touch can lend an element of bonding unlike any other connection. Placing a hand on someone's shoulder or grasping someone's hand can speak volumes.

Information

Patients want to know what's going on. Make every effort to keep them informed and involved in their care. Give thorough explanations about tests, treatments, and medications. Let them know that you want to keep them informed and invite their questions. Put things in writing whenever possible. Patient education has always been a vital nursing function.

Respect

Respect is a basic need that is often lacking in the patient-provider interaction. The chapter on standards reviewed behavior that demonstrates respect, including making eye contact, talking to patients rather than over them, and using their name. But the real core of respect falls back to your personal beliefs. If you don't feel everyone is worthy of respect, it will be difficult to fake the associated behaviors.

Privacy

No other profession invades an individual's privacy like health care. Patients are stripped down and expected to share some of the most intimate details of their lives with health care providers. Their physical and psychological conditions become an open book the moment patients enter the system. There are a few actions that can help demonstrate your respect for patient privacy. They include the following:

- Knock when entering the room. Even when the door stands open, knocking sends a signal that you are seeking permission to enter the patient's personal space. Ask permission to enter the room.
- Draw privacy curtains or close doors before asking the patient to expose any body parts. Do this when helping patients out of bed as well. Hospital gowns were never designed for modesty. Even the slightest movements can cause embarrassing exposure.
- Contain discussions with patients to their rooms or a private conference area. Nurses are so accustomed to talking with patients about bodily functions that many tend to forget how personal these topics are for patients. I have heard nurses stop patients in the hall and ask about bowel movements, gas, and vaginal discharge. Never, never, never discuss bodily functions in the hall or within earshot of other patients or visitors. Even if no one is around, talking about these things in the hall implies a lack of respect for patient privacy.
- Respect confidentiality at all times. There is never an excuse for talking about patients with anyone without a direct need to know. Even if names are not used, talking over "cases" around the cafeteria table or in the elevator is inexcusable. Family members, visitors, and even vendors who observe these conversations make assumptions about the organization's commitment to confidentiality.
- Whenever it is necessary to ask patients personal questions, let them know why you are asking. Tell them what it has to do

with the assessment or treatment, then tell them the information will be kept in strict confidence. Doing so helps patients understand the relevance and reassures them of privacy.

Attitude

People often assume that they're born with a positive attitude or they're not, and there's nothing that they can do about it. That assumption is wrong. Attitude is totally within the realm of your control. It is completely internal. Although external events are not within your control, your reaction to the events is completely within your control. I have never met anyone who sees himself or herself as negative. Most negative people I have known are oblivious to their demeanor as well as the impact it has on others. But bad attitudes are everywhere and, left unchecked, can destroy an organization like a virulent disease. Chronic complaining, criticizing, and looking for fault in others are the trademarks of the classic bad attitude. A self-assessment is a good place to start, but sometimes it takes another person to point out how others perceive you.

Smile. The social smile is one of our first indications that we are connecting with those around us. Even for an infant six weeks old, the social smile triggers a huge jump in maternal-infant bonding. Throughout life, a smile is one of the most basic gestures of welcome, kindness, and acceptance, yet it is quickly dropped during busy shifts and time of stress. Patients look for a smile as a gesture of care and comfort. Many of us (myself included) don't smile when we're deep in thought. It takes conscious effort to remind yourself to smile at times.

Victim thinking can be lethal to positive results. No one likes to be a victim, yet often our thoughts and attitudes make us into victims. It takes self-awareness to recognize victim thinking and conscious effort to stop it. What is victim thinking? Here are some of the classics: "They don't give us enough staff." "They don't understand." "They expect too much." "They don't give a damn about us little people." "They only care about the money." "They don't know our patients like we do."

Who are *they* anyway? My simple definition is this. The word *they* is a collective noun representing the oppressive force that is robbing the nurse of control. *They* could be administration. *They* could be the insurance company. *They* could be coworkers, other departments, or nurses working other shifts. But somehow *they* are always hovering and threatening to make the nurses' lives hell. Ask yourself this simple question: "Am I part of the problem or part of the solution?" Chronic complaining about circumstances won't change them. By choosing to be part of the solution, you are breaking out of the victim role. You'll be surprised to see how liberating that can be.

Moments of Truth

Each of us has moments of truth when we choose one path over another. Every day presents us with countless opportunities to perform acceptably or exceptionally, but the choice is always ours alone. When a patient needs to be turned, you do it with skill and care. That's acceptable. But when you add a one-minute back massage and comforting conversation, it becomes exceptional. If things get quiet at the end of your shift, do you spend the few extra minutes chatting with coworkers or choose to do one more thing for a patient that would make him or her more comfortable? I have found that nurses who regularly take the exceptional path during these moments of truth find much greater satisfaction with their work.

Applause, Applause

Wouldn't it be great if you were recognized for every act of exceptional customer service? You can be. Do it yourself. You can't rely on others to observe and comment on your performance throughout the day. But you know when you've done a good job. So congratulate yourself. It's important to give yourself credit for extra effort. Doing so throughout the day can help to boost your spirits.

Don't Forget Your Other Customers

Although patients have been the focus of the majority of this chapter, physicians and coworkers are important customers too. Unfortunately, we tend to slight our coworkers more than any other customer group. Housekeepers, maintenance workers, dietary aides, and volunteers are essential members of the health care team and are as deserving of our respect and positive attitude as the patients. Discourteous behavior toward any coworker is unacceptable. Yet I could cite at least a hundred examples of rude and disrespectful behavior by nurses toward other staff members. Somehow there seems to be an assumption that people not directly involved in patient care are not as important as we are. That sentiment is communicated clearly by behavior. In other words, actions speak louder than words.

During focus groups with employees, I tried to identify what staff wanted from coworkers. The number one thing mentioned was respect. They want to know that their work is valued by others and to know that they are an important part of the team. Review the guidelines presented on the previous pages in this chapter, but this time with your coworkers in mind. Identify at least one action in each area that you could take to become more service-minded with them.

Phone Etiquette

Entire books and training courses have been devoted to the topic of telephone skills. I don't intend to go into that depth here, but I want to point out that many of your coworker or physician contacts occur over the phone. In even the briefest conversations, when you pick up the phone, you become the face and voice of the organization. Treat phone contacts with the same regard as you would face-to-face contacts. The following list offers a few pointers for improving phone skills:

- Always greet the caller with "Hello," "Good morning," "Good afternoon," or "Good evening."
- State your name and the department.
- Ask, "How may I help you?"
- Speak clearly and slowly, especially when reciting numbers.
- Smile. Even on the phone, a smile can be "heard."
- Recap the conversation briefly.
- End the conversation with a polite closure and goodbye. "Thank you for calling. Goodbye."

I have worked with some people who are incredibly compassionate and caring with patients but become aloof and even rude with coworkers. I've never quite understood the Dr. Jekyll and Mr. Hyde performance, but I'm convinced that it persists because intolerable behavior is tolerated. Each of us has a responsibility to confront coworkers who are rude or abrupt with others. It's not an easy task but is essential if we hope to improve customer service and, hence, satisfaction. If you are not sure how your coworkers perceive you, ask them. Their feedback may surprise you and help you set some specific goals.

Summary

None of the techniques outlined in this chapter are rocket science. They are, however, some of the basic skills that can shape customer perceptions of nurses. Members of the nursing profession are fortunate to have so many opportunities to shape perceptions of the health care experience. Improving perceptions requires that we first understand the needs of our customers and behave in a manner that exceeds their expectations. But the changes needed must happen by design. Improving skills takes conscious effort and consistency. By following the guidelines presented in this chapter, nurses can raise the level of customer service from good to great!

CHAPTER TEN

Measuring Results

Objectives

After completing this chapter the reader will:

- Recognize the importance of measuring satisfaction among specific customer groups

- Have the tools for measuring results using qualitative and quantitative methods

- Identify methods for communicating results to stakeholder groups

After training, communicating, and rewarding, it's time to see how well your efforts have been working. In chapter 4 you learned the importance of creating baseline data on patient, employee, and physician satisfaction. This chapter will help you gauge the improvements you have made since the first steps of customer service implementation. Although it is always desirable to be able to quantify your results, there are softer indicators of success that should not be overlooked. This chapter will help you identify both the quantitative and qualitative results of your efforts.

Back to the Beginning—Quantifiable Data

Although quantifying data may feel like the end of the process, it isn't. As with any quality or process improvement plan, the measurement step is not the end but part of the cycle that will lead you to your next set of plans.

In our organization the quantifiable patient satisfaction measurement is ongoing, so we are able to monitor trends monthly or quarterly. Employee and physician satisfaction, however, is conducted much less frequently. Assuming that you have collected baseline information for each of these groups as instructed in chapter 4, you will probably want to wait at least 6 to 12 months before reassessing. Not only do you need time to show results, but the survey process can be laborious and time-consuming for the participants who may not take kindly to frequent surveys.

Patient Satisfaction

At this point, it's appropriate to compare the data from your baseline patient satisfaction with the most current data. Look for organizationwide as well as department-specific trends. Watertown set specific goals for the percent of responses falling in the "excellent" category. Many of the customer service action plans targeted behaviors that would move them from good to excellent scores. We also set goals for the percent of respondents that indicated they are very likely to recommend our hospital or clinic to others. This is a good indicator of loyalty as well as positive word of mouth.

Keep track of the number of positive and negative comments on the surveys as well. This helps provide another view of patient perceptions.

Unsolicited complaints are another way of measuring results. Our hospital and clinics keep close tabs on the number, nature, and source of unsolicited complaints. We found that in the first two quarters following the customer service training, we had a significant decline in the number of unsolicited complaints.

Employee Satisfaction

Ideally, a second measurement of employee satisfaction will show improvement from your baseline. (Remember to use the same measurement tools you used to gain your baseline data for a valid comparison.) Look especially for stark contrasts in satisfaction from one department to another that may indicate some issues in management and leadership. As with the patient satisfaction surveys, tabulate the number of positive and negative comments from employees as well.

Physician Satisfaction

Chances are good that physicians were targeted in several of the departmental action plans. If the plans were successfully implemented, it is likely that you will see some improvement in physician satisfaction when compared with the initial baseline data.

Sharing the Results

Communicating satisfaction results to key stakeholder groups is an important part of your overall success. It's not just OK to brag, it's necessary. Employees need to know that their efforts are paying off, administrators and board members will want to know about quality improvement efforts, and, finally, the managed care companies are often looking at patient satisfaction scores in clinics and hospitals.

Going public with satisfaction scores can be a real boost for public image and employee morale (assuming that the scores are good). We periodically publish data summaries in our internal newsletter and external newsletter. Individual departments should be encouraged to post scores on bulletin boards and discuss them at unit meetings.

Presenting the scores at medical staff meetings, at management information meetings, and in employee updates offers opportunities for participants to ask questions. This can be an important part of building buy-in.

Qualitative Indicators of Success

Although it's important to measure and monitor satisfaction through quantifiable methods, qualitative indicators of success should be recognized as well. Ignoring or minimizing these softer indicators could be a mistake. These are the little changes that make our jobs more enjoyable. They are the milestones that tell us we are moving from the old ways of thinking into a culture of service excellence. For me, it's the little things that, when added up, speak volumes about our organization's progress.

Small Steps Will Take You Miles

When you are the person leading a customer service effort, there may be times when you wonder if anything is getting through to anyone, so it's important to watch for the little victories that are the true indicators of success. Since this is an ongoing process, it often becomes difficult to spot the "Olympic moments" that refresh your spirit. Keep your eyes open for those moments when you see evidence that the message is getting through. Watch and observe how your colleagues have taken the message to heart. Comment and compliment them when you see exemplary behavior, but also take the time to congratulate yourself for persisting at crafting the new culture.

Olympic Moments

Following are a few Olympic moments from Watertown Memorial Hospital. The gold medallists are the individuals who took the initiative to act on behalf of the organization even when it wasn't in the job description. While none of these acts in and of themselves would win a Nobel Prize or even the Malcom Baldridge award for quality improvement, they are the little steps that affirmed that someone was listening and taking the message to heart. I call them Olympic moments because, like the athletes who represent our country in competition, it all comes back to the individuals who create a winning reputation for our organization.

"Don" from maintenance used to go about his business at the hospital and pretty much stick to his business and nothing else. That's in part because of the training and example that had been set for him at the outset. His job was to stick to maintenance. But during a renovation project in radiology, patients had to be temporarily relocated to the surgeon's lounge for ultrasound. The setup had looked pretty good to the department staff and the architect, so they proceeded as planned. Don was passing through the area while working on the renovation and voiced his concern to the manager that patients didn't have enough privacy. He then made a suggestion about how he could help them correct the situation. "I just knew it wasn't right. I wouldn't want to be the patient having a test done where someone could walk by and see me."

I wonder if Don would have spoken up in the past. He may have wanted to, but if the culture didn't support critical thinking regardless of one's title, he may have passed up the opportunity. Even worse, he may have gone back to his own department and commented about "those dopes in radiology" and left it at that. I wouldn't have even heard about Don's suggestion but for a routine report at the monthly board of directors meeting.

While updating the board on the renovation progress, our VP of nursing mentioned the privacy snafu that had been spotted and corrected by someone from maintenance. It didn't take long for me to trace it back to Don. I made it a point to tell him in front of his peers that his story had been shared with the board and thanked him for speaking up.

Marv Kaufmann is a newer member of our hospital auxiliary. A retired marketing professional, Marv is a wellspring of enthusiasm. He truly enjoys his work and often goes above and beyond the call of duty when working at the information desk or escorting patients. Although Marv arrived with a very clear understanding of customer service, he wanted to do something that would help other volunteers to understand the importance of the little extras. One day he appeared in the volunteer director's office and simply handed her this note and said, "I went home from the hospital last night so inspired, I just had to write this down":

> As I prepare for each time I volunteer, I do so with one over-arching goal: to make every time an event. I'm a firm believer in tradition, but my goal is to add something extra to some visitor or patient's discharge beyond what is expected. I'm eager to share the excitement of flowers, mail, or going home with people of all ages. I take advantage of each situation to share and sell that "blue jacket" and Watertown Memorial Hospital. This sharing with others offers a special experience you cannot find elsewhere. It can expand your horizons and energize your soul, even as it relaxes and refreshes your mind and body. It's like giving your spirit a workout and a massage all at once.

Marv didn't have to write this message. He didn't have to share it. But Marv followed his heart and shared his passion with others. We not only thanked him for his prose, we published it in the volunteer newsletter and on the back of the awards dinner program.

Sharon is an assistant in the human resources department. Having been with the organization for more than 20 years in various capacities, Sharon has pretty much seen it all. When we first met, Sharon worked in payroll. In order to process the payroll, Sharon required very specific details on time cards. Not being a detail-oriented person, I would be summoned to Sharon's office periodically and gently reminded that I should not turn in my departments' time cards without more specific details. She patiently showed me the correct way and I invariably forgot and sent in incomplete ones week after week. I don't want to say I was the one who pushed her over the edge, but not long after I started, Sharon transferred from payroll to human resources. Again Sharon was in charge of the reams of papers necessary to process any change in personnel. And invariably I messed up. About the time Sharon transferred, we completed the first round of organizationwide customer service training. I don't know if I just wore her down, or if customer service training helped something to click, but Sharon changed her approach with me. One day she called me and said, "I know you have your hands full and that you are in the process of hiring staff for the new clinic. To make the paperwork a little easier for you, I'm sending over copies of M-100s (the infamous essential paper that turns an ordinary citizen into a WMH employee with the stroke of a pen). All you have to do is sign and return them; I've filled out all the rest." An Olympic moment. Sharon realized the intensity of my workload and stepped in to do what she could to make the job go smoother.

In the past Sharon may have persisted in trying to train me about details that would have continually escaped me as I grappled with bigger issues of business development. But Sharon got it. Something clicked when she started seeing me as a customer. Eureka!

Sharon had another Olympic moment that only the two of us shared, but for me it was evidence that the team was finally moving in the same direction. She called one day to say that a journal article about building a service culture had been circulated to department managers. She said, "When I read this I thought of you. This is everything you have been saying to us since the day you arrived. I have to admit that I blew you off in the beginning. Yeah, yeah, this customer service is just another fad. I thought, 'I'll think about that stuff when I have time.' But you never wavered from day one. You have persisted in helping us to think about it every day and in everything we do. I know I have changed, and I really think a lot of others have too."

At that moment I knew what it might feel like to be Bruce Jenner's coach in the 1970s. I wasn't the champion, but perhaps my coaching was helping to build champions. For most of us working in health care, our days are full and getting fuller. Keeping up with all the changes and volumes of information can seem insurmountable. It's vital for leaders and coaches to take the time to spot the little strides that are carrying your team to the final goal. Then stop and congratulate yourself. While the journey isn't over, at least you know you are on the right track.

Who Else Should See Your Results?

Foremost among the other interested parties who should see your measures of success are payers, board members, employers, and donors.

- *Payers*—Many managed care organizations and insurance companies are looking at report cards to indicate how well their members are being served. Use your data to demonstrate that your organization is concerned and attentive to its members.
- *Board members*—Quality improvement is often at the core of board focus. The customer service champion should plan to conduct at least one customer service update for the board each year. Tell the board about the process and show it the trends observed.
- *Employers*—The largest purchasers of health care services are employers. Like the payers cited above, employers want to know that their employees have options for high-quality health care services locally. If your organization has a newsletter for employers, consider dedicating an issue each year to spotlight satisfaction. If you don't have such a newsletter, consider

sending out a direct mail piece on the subject. It could be as simple as a letter or as detailed as a full report.

- *Donors*—Many health care organizations are the beneficiaries of regular financial donations from community members. Philanthropists who give donations to your hospital or system want to know that they are giving to a winning organization. If you have a regular publication for donors, include a report at least once a year summarizing satisfaction data. Make sure to state the organization's commitment to customer service as well as the core values and standards. Showing the satisfaction results in the context of the commitment can reassure the donors that their money is going to a progressive organization.

Summary

Measuring your results brings you back to the beginning of the customer service process. Although comparison with baseline data may give the illusion of the end, you are now at the point of reassessing priorities and reformulating action plans. It is important to summarize the data from all the sources and again identify the strengths, weaknesses, opportunities, and threats (see chapter 5). In doing so, you will have a new baseline from which you can develop further action plans.

Continuing this process on a scheduled basis will ensure that you are keeping the customer service focus throughout the organization. Progress will not happen by itself. You will need to continually reassess, plan, and implement new steps in order to continue raising the bar. But once you have made a full cycle through the process, it will become easier to implement the necessary steps to keep the initiative going.

Conclusion

The process outlined in this book is one that has been successfully implemented at Watertown Area Health Services.

Although our results are far from perfect, the steps outlined have provided a logical, pragmatic progression toward our customer service goals. We continue to make consistent progress.

By following the process described here, you will have the necessary tools for implementing a grassroots approach to customer service excellence in your own organization.

The keys to success are consistency, persistence, optimism, and, above all, support from the top administration. There will be times throughout this process when you wonder if anyone else is on board and still other times when the small Olympic moments and satisfaction ratings reaffirm your faith in your colleagues. Persistence and commitment will bear fruit in the form of positive results.

Beginning with your statement of core values, followed by standards development and training sessions, a successful initiative requires a solid foundation. But none of these steps can be accomplished without teamwork from individuals throughout the organization. In order to craft a truly grassroots effort you will need to gain support from all levels and disciplines. Although time-consuming, the results from this process are extremely gratifying. Involving multidisciplinary team members creates a groundswell of support for the initiative.

As health care organizations, we have a unique opportunity to serve others during some of life's most trying and vulnerable moments. By placing customer service at the forefront of our daily activities, we will be improving the patient experience through care, compassion, and unwavering courtesy. There is no other segment of the service industry that holds this level of responsibility. And, therefore, no other that can reap the level of personal satisfaction for a job well done. Whether measured by market share, quantifiable satisfaction scores, or employee morale, a grassroots approach to customer service will help you create an environment where patients want to be treated, where physicians want to practice, and where employees want to work.

Index